Managing Drugs in Sport

As ongoing high-profile drug scandals have demonstrated, sports organisations rarely have a coherent strategy to manage the role and relationship their sport has with different types of drugs (from alcohol to supplements to prescription drugs to doping). This important and timely book argues that drug control-led integrity management of sport is more than an ideological battle around doping. The relationship sport has with the drugs industry has become a much broader management problem. The breadth of the problem compels stakeholders in sport (including athletes, coaches, fans, public servants and sports managers) to understand better the issues in pursuit of effective strategies and responses.

Drawing on cutting-edge management theory, this book explores the dilemma of drugs in sport. It introduces the policy and business contexts that have shaped responses to this issue and examines its significance to sport and integrity management, including human resource management, marketing and risk management. It discusses practical management concerns, such as working with scientists and anti-doping organisations, and offers clear recommendations for the future management of sports integrity.

The first book to offer a complete framework for a drugs management strategy for sport, *Managing Drugs in Sport* is essential reading for all advanced students, researchers and practitioners working in sport management, sport business, sport policy, sport governance and business ethics.

Jason Mazanov is a Senior Lecturer in the School of Business at UNSW-Canberra, Australia. He is a registered psychologist whose primary work has been explaining drug use, particularly the use of performance enhancing substances. He is a founding editor of the scholarly journal *Performance Enhancement and Health*, has contributed to numerous published works on the management of drugs in sport in the peer-review literature and media and has taught organisational behaviour, leadership, human resource management and public sector management to the Masters level.

Routledge Research in Sport Business and Management

Available in this series:

Managing Drugs in Sport

Jason Mazanov

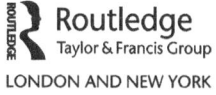

Routledge
Taylor & Francis Group

LONDON AND NEW YORK

First published 2017
by Routledge
2 Park Square, Milton Park, Abingdon, Oxon OX14 4RN

and by Routledge
711 Third Avenue, New York, NY 10017

First issued in paperback 2018

Routledge is an imprint of the Taylor & Francis Group, an informa business

British Library Cataloguing-in-Publication Data
A catalogue record for this book is available from the British
Library

Library of Congress Cataloging in Publication Data
Names: Mazanov, Jason, author.
Title: Managing drugs in sport / Jason Mazanov.
Description: Milton Park, Abingdon, Oxon ; New York, NY :
Routledge, 2016. |
Series: Routledge research in sport business and management |
Includes bibliographical references and index.
Identifiers: LCCN 2016019399| ISBN 9781138803480 (hardback) |
ISBN 9781315753690 (ebook)
Subjects: LCSH: Doping in sports. | Athletes–Drug use. | Sports
medicine–Moral and ethical aspects.
Classification: LCC RC1230 .M3758 2016 | DDC 362.29/088796–dc23
LC record available at https://lccn.loc.gov/2016019399

ISBN 13: 978-1-138-59518-7 (pbk)
ISBN 13: 978-1-138-80348-0 (hbk)

Typeset in Sabon
by Wearset Ltd, Boldon, Tyne and Wear

This book is dedicated to the late Professor Peter Hall

Contents

Acknowledgements

The book is dedicated to the memory of Professor Peter Hall. Professor Hall gave me my start as a fully-fledged academic, and took responsibility for helping me build that career. Professor Hall did so because it was, to his mind, the right thing to do. Professor Hall was a person of remarkable integrity, and one of the few genuine scholars I have had the privilege of meeting or working with. I hope that I can pay forward even a little of what he taught me.

Throughout this project I have enjoyed the support of a wide range of people. From among my many colleagues in the world of academia, two have been particularly influential throughout this project. First, the unfailing rigour and good sense of Twan Huybers provided much-needed constancy. Second, Norm O'Reilly gave me the confidence to both commence and complete this project.

Outside the world of academia, I have drawn inspiration from the lyrics of Fear Factory (in all their forms), and their challenge to think about the symbiotic relationship between man and machine. And their music was a good way to exit the fog that comes with writing a book!

Finally, I hope my family finds the investment we have made into this project worthwhile. And so, it is to my sweet bride that this project is truly indebted – onwards and upwards, my love!

Part I

Context

Chapter 1

Managing integrity in sport

The case of drug control

Modern sport is premised on an assumption that sport is inherently good and pure, that the inherent goodness and purity is transmitted to those associated with sport, and that sport enhances individuals and communities (Coakley, 2015, p. 404). Coakley's 'great sport myth' is borne out in practice, demonstrated by sport creating opportunities for social mobility, allowing nations to unite behind extraordinary athletes in times of adversity, driving technological innovation and inspiring people to test the limits of human performance. However, the great sport myth is also contradicted by the apparent exploitation of children and the poor, the marginalisation of women, and athletes being sacrificed for the sake of national prestige. The attempt to preserve the assumed goodness and purity of sport has seen both sporting institutions and governments engage in extraordinary management practices – giving rise to the need to manage the 'integrity of sport'.

Management of the integrity of sport is an attempt to manage the trust relationship between stakeholders in organisational contexts (Kaptein, 1999). That is, sports consumers (e.g. fans, gamblers, sponsors, broadcasters and governments) trust that producers (e.g. athletes and sports managers) have practised sport in line with a combination of rules-based and values-based expectations (Maesschlak & Vanden Auweele, 2010). For example, Treagus, Cover and Beasley's (2011) review summarises expectations about the integrity of sport as 'respect for oneself and others, moral responsibility and accountability' (p. 5). Australia's National Integrity for Sport Unit (NISU) defines integrity as 'fair and honest performances ... unaffected by external influences' and 'positive conduct ... which enhances the standing of the sporting contest and of sport overall'. Applied to sport, threats to the perceived integrity of sport emerge when there is a violation of the trust placed in producers to preserve the inherent goodness and purity. From this point of view, integrity management is understood negatively rather than positively, as it is most apparent when it is absent. Integrity management in sport seeks to prevent violations of expectations in the production process and to respond effectively should violations occur.

Across the pantheon of threats to the integrity of sport, drugs and match fixing are widely understood to be the two greatest threats. Of these two threats, the attempt to manage the integrity of sport through managing drugs in sport makes drugs the single most dominant threat in the eyes of sporting institutions and governments. Sporting institutions see threats to the integrity of sport arising from drugs as diminishing the value of their products, whether violating norms of 'fairness' in sport, as a function of the consumer base (e.g. attracting new consumers through junior sport), attracting free labour to events (e.g. volunteers), or revenue from ticket sales, broadcasting, advertising or merchandise. Governments see drug threats to the integrity of sport as diminishing the assumed social benefits of sport, such as public health (e.g. obesity) or sports development programmes. The significance of the threat posed by drugs in sport has moved both sporting institutions and governments to a level of international co-operation unseen in many other areas of international relations. The international effort to manage the integrity of sport through managing drugs commands significant ongoing investment, with an estimated global cost of at least US$500 million per annum (Maennig, 2014).

The aim of this book is to build the understanding of managing integrity in sport by examining the management of drugs in sport. In doing so, an assessment can be made about whether the attempt to manage drugs has protected the integrity of sport. The analysis and assessment can also be used to draw conclusions about managing the integrity of sport, and managing integrity more broadly.

Managing drugs and integrity: corporate social responsibility

A core theme in this book is that the management of drugs in sport goes well beyond anti-doping. While anti-doping has become the dominant ideology and discourse when it comes to managing drugs in sport, it is incorrect to equate anti-doping with drug management. For example, the anti-doping policy has no bearing on abuse of alcohol by fans at sporting events, or athlete misuse of prescription drugs. Sporting institutions have an obligation to broader society to manage their relationship with drugs broadly, rather than one form of drug consumption (see Chapter 2). Moreover, there is an obligation to consider how management of drugs impacts beyond the private interests of sporting institutions (Carroll, 1979), such as the impact upon public policy or social issues (Walker & Parent, 2010). Smith and Westerbeek (2007) warn that sport must be aware of its ideological positioning within societies given its significant role in both public policy (e.g. health initiatives) and as a vehicle to respond to broader social issues (e.g. drug education).

Given sport's responsibility to society when managing drugs, it is perhaps surprising that the management of drugs in sport has been a conspicuous absentee from the broader discussion of corporate social responsibility (CSR) in sport (see Paramio-Salcines, Babiak, & Walters, 2013). Discussions on CSR and sport have focused on activities that promote the 'great sport myth' such as how sport helps society address poverty, education or public health (Breitbarth, Walzel, Anagnostopoulos, & van Eekeren, 2015) rather than issues that might contradict the myth by addressing discrimination against women, exploitation of children or hooliganism (cf. Babiak, 2010; Godfrey, 2009). Where such issues are discussed, they are usually discussed in terms of protecting brands from product harm crises or 'greenwashing' scandal (e.g. Godfrey, 2009; Levermore, 2013; Levermore & Moore, 2015; Sheth & Babiak, 2010). As a consequence, it is appropriate to determine the extent of sport's responsibility to manage drugs.

Analysis of sport's responsibility using the wide array of conceptual models offered by CSR scholars can be a daunting and difficult choice. Acknowledging the breadth of debate over the different approaches to and understanding of CSR, the approach taken to evaluate the nature and extent of the responsibility that members of the sports sector assume for managing drugs needs to cut across the debate. Dahlsrud's (2008) analysis of definitions provides a set of five dimensions (stakeholder, social, economic, voluntariness and environment) that captures what is generally understood to constitute CSR, which is sufficient for the current purposes. Importantly, Dahlsrud's five dimensions offer the flexibility to explore the issues associated with CSR, sport and drugs necessary to assess the breadth of sport's responsibilities in relation to managing drugs.

Stakeholders

Organisations which make up the sports sector are mutually reliant upon those who practise sport – the athletes (Mazanov, 2014). The practice of sport leads to sports consumption. For the purposes of the argument, sports consumption is divided into those with an interest in organising events that enable sport to be practised, creating stakeholders *internal* to sports production (e.g. athletes, coaches, medical practitioners and sports administrators), and those who watch events, creating stakeholders *external* to sports production (e.g. broadcasting, merchandising and regulation).

Stakeholders internal to sports production

The governance mechanisms that attempt to reconcile the interests of athletes and stakeholders internal to sports production have a significant influence on the management of drugs in sport. Indeed, governance was singled out as the most important reason underlying the supplements scandal that engulfed the Essendon Football Club through the 2013–2015 Australian Football League seasons (Court of Arbitration for Sport, 2016; Phat, Birt, Turner, & Fenech, 2015). Elements within the club acted independently, and were assessed on objectively measurable outcomes rather than ongoing and regular review of compliance with policy and procedures. As a result, the narrow interests of a minority of stakeholders compromised the club. While corporatisation of sport has sought to overcome such governance problems by improving transparency arrangements (e.g. Chappelet, 2011), the ongoing claims of corruption at the highest levels of managing drugs in sport, such as the systematic concealment of doping in professional cycling (e.g. Lance Armstrong) and athletics (e.g. Russia) and the failure to regulate the supplements industry (Pipe & Ayotte, 2002; Swann, 2015), suggest there is some way to go.

Where sport formalises relationships with drug manufacturers (e.g. supplying drugs to athletes), there is a duty of care to athletes to ensure that the drugs in question do what they claim (see Outram & Stewart, 2015). While some drugs have beneficial effects (e.g. creatine; Beduschi, 2003), there is often no evidence to support the claims made about the sports specific effects of drugs, ranging from supplements (e.g. 'natural' testosterone enhancers; Qureshi, Naughton, & Petróczi, 2014) to prescription drugs (e.g. human growth hormone; López, 2013). The dubious nature of the claims can lead to potentially harmful drug consumption that could otherwise be avoided. This was a key point in the Essendon case, with the club sanctioned by government workplace health and safety where the introduction of drugs led to a failure to provide a safe working environment (Longbottom, 2016).

Stakeholders external to sports production

External stakeholders who watch sporting events create markets with both direct and derived demand for sports production and consumption (Borland & Macdonald, 2003). This includes selling access to sporting events (e.g. broadcasters, sponsors and advertisers) or access to merchandising (e.g. equipment, apparel, collectables and mediated content). These external stakeholders influence management of drugs in sport in pursuit of their private interests (cf. Crompton, 2014, pp. 420–423). For example, pressure from sponsors to get 'star players' on-field can drive the misuse of prescription substances such as analgesics or sleeping tablets (Anderson & Jackson, 2013; Orchard et al., 2010). Off-field events can also be problematic, such as players feeling obligated to be seen consuming a sponsor's alcoholic product, and doing so to excess (O'Brien & Kypri, 2008). Media organisations with a stake in sports organisations may manufacture drug scandals to sell content that ends athletes' careers (cf. Connor & Mazanov, 2010; Frenger, Emrich, & Pitsch, 2013). The CSR agenda indicates that sport has a responsibility to protect athletes from such coercive pressures (Smith & Westerbeek, 2007).

The interest in and implications arising from sports consumption means that governments are a stakeholder in both sports production and consumption due to the implications for health (e.g. healthcare implications of sports injuries), revenue (e.g. taxation), gambling (e.g. policing illegal betting) and advertising (e.g. tobacco and alcohol). Governments and other public organisations also bring significant pressure to bear on how they want drug issues in sport to be managed. For example, as argued in Chapter 3, public agencies put significant pressure on sporting organisations to find alternatives to cigarette and alcohol sponsorship in the interest of public health, with some countries making the practice illegal. The CSR element here is to ensure that the private interests of sport (e.g. revenue and participation) are managed relative to the public interests of governments (e.g. public health, policing and taxation). Deference to public interests is appropriate under favourable financial circumstances (Carroll, 1979). For example, increasing revenue from media rights may see sport able to prioritise its relationship with public health over that of alcohol sponsorship, as occurred when Australian University Sport (2009) cited public health interests as a driving reason behind the decision to divest itself of alcohol sponsorship entirely.

Social

CSR seeks to preserve both the internal value of sport to producers and consumers (e.g. sporting capital; Rowe, 2015) and the external value of sport to broader society (e.g. social capital; Stewart & Smith, 2014). Rowe (2015) argues that the internal value of sport is generated by its impact on psychological well-being (e.g. self-esteem and identity), social well-being (e.g. connection with community) and physiological well-being (e.g. physical competency). This means both producers and consumers must be concerned with the internal welfare of sport, such as establishing and defending rules set up to enable sports events to occur. The CSR agenda and managing drugs in sport converge when considering the welfare of the communities directly involved in sport relative to sports-related drug consumption impacting upon psychological, social and physiological well-being. Sport can become a bastion to ameliorate the impact of drug misuse and abuse in wider society (e.g. alcohol or crack) by preserving the internal value of sport for the community. While sport has been involved in such efforts, they appear to be haphazard or opportunistic to the point they could be considered 'greenwashing'. The principles of CSR indicate generating sporting capital through social capital by ameliorating drug misuse and abuse should be achieved through sustained institutional responses, such as the Australian 'Good Sports' and 'Be the Influence' campaigns.

Sport also has external value to broader society by creating connections across communities (Nicholson & Hoye, 2008). Sporting capital translates into social capital when the values associated with drug use in sport are adopted by other elements in society. For example, anti-doping appears to be shaping the way people understand the role of human enhancing technology across competitive non-sporting contexts (e.g. academia; Partridge, Lucke, & Hall, 2014) and is becoming a model for regulating other behaviours that compromise well-established principles of civil and criminal procedures (Smith, 2014). Sport has a responsibility to ensure that the values it projects promote rather than diminish the evolution of society. For example, questions have been raised whether the anti-doping system is inhibiting the use of performance enhancing substances that might otherwise improve the quality of life for individuals, and the economic competitiveness and prosperity of nations (Beddington *et al.*, 2008).

Economic

In terms of the economic domain of CSR, the management of drugs in sport becomes a question of its impact on commercial viability. In the first instance, the approach taken by sport should ensure that the benefits arising from a particular form of drug management exceed the costs. The dominance of the anti-doping ideology brought with it the conventional wisdom that sports specific drugs diminish consumer demand, and ultimately the commercial viability of sport (e.g. Carstairs, 2003; Møller & Dimeo, 2014; Solberg, Hanstad, & Thøring, 2010). While drug-related scandal can clearly have an impact on some aspects of commercial viability in sport (e.g. the loss of revenues to Lance Armstrong, Barry Bonds and Michael Phelps), it is incorrect to assume these effects extrapolate across drug types and across sporting institutions (e.g. recreational sport).

The anxiety that drugs diminish consumer demand may be misplaced. For example, the average twenty-first century elite Olympian, world athletics championship athlete or FIFA World Cup player competes with 2.5–3.0 substances in their system (Tscholl, Junge, & Dvorak, 2008; Tscholl, Alonso, Dollé, Junge, & Dvorak, 2010; Tsitsimpikou *et al.*, 2009) with little discernible impact on revenue trajectories for any of those events. Models identifying the independent contribution of different types of drug consumption (e.g. performance enhancement, recovery or injury rehabilitation) on revenue in sport are yet to be reported. The evidence available suggests drug scandal temporarily reduces consumer demand for broadcast or attendance, even for professional cycling (Buechel, Emrich, & Pohlkamp, 2014; Van Reeth, 2013). For example, the 8 per cent drop in Major League Baseball home game attendance following a drug scandal breaking disappeared within 15 days (Cisyk & Courty, 2015). Thus, the anxiety that drugs diminish consumer demand appears to be misplaced.

Drugs can play a valuable role in protecting and growing the commercial viability of sport. Drawing on Mottram's (2015) discussion of the uses for drugs in sporting contexts, drugs can expand the participation base of the market by making sport safer (e.g. arresting training-based depression of the immune system), improving access (e.g. beta-agonists allowing those with asthma to participate) and prolonging participation by protecting athlete health from sports-related illnesses or injuries (e.g. Masters athletes) (cf. Marcora, 2016). The correlation between participation and consumption (Bennett, Ferreira, Lee, & Polite, 2009; Summers & Johnson, 1999) means that a larger participation base also means a larger consumer base. At the elite level, drugs can produce spectacles of interest to consumers (e.g. world records) and therefore sponsors and advertisers. Managing drug consumption therefore represents a potentially valuable tool to both preserve and grow the commercial viability of sport with regards to the consumer base, so long as the benefits exceed the costs that arise from the responsibility arising from such consumption. Where costs exceed the benefits, sport may be better to conclude its relationship with those drugs.

Voluntariness

This domain accounts for sport's responsibility to manage drugs in a way that reflects the communities it comes from in terms of values (ethics) beyond both the intention and letter of local laws. Note that this discussion is focused on establishing the case for managing drugs in sport relative to CSR rather than discussing anti-doping specifically. See Chapter 6 for a discussion on the ethical implications of anti-doping.

Sport has a responsibility to manage drugs given its privileged status and significant influence on society (e.g. the relationship between sport and health) for the reasons outlined under the social dimension. Mazanov (2014) argues that the fundamental basis for sport's management of drugs arises from its obligations to reflect drug control in broader society, such as the responsibility to protect participants (Smith & Westerbeek, 2007). To demonstrate this, Mazanov uses examples of:

- an amphetamine-crazed hockey player attacking another player with their stick,
- exploitation by parents giving children human growth hormone in the hope they will be tall or heavy enough for a particular sport,
- using powerful pharmaceuticals without medical supervision, and
- worker safety arising from the implications of alcohol use in motor sports.

These examples can be used to establish the need for managing drugs across organisational contexts generally, and sport specifically. From this point of view, where sport enjoys the benefits of society it also has an obligation to voluntarily promote drug control beyond its legal obligations to be consistent with the values of the society it comes from.

Whether sport voluntarily changes its management of drugs comes into focus in the context of changing rules and norms around the role of drugs in society. For example, the legalisation of marijuana in several jurisdictions raises questions about whether sport should reflect the values of those societies or impose its own values around marijuana. As noted in discussion of the social dimension, the resistance to or acceptance of local laws and values means sport can influence local laws and values. In this instance, sport must consider whether its acceptance or resistance drives sporting interests at the expense of community interests, or contributes to the overall welfare of local and global communities. Thus, sport has the opportunity to engage in 'good corporate citizenship' through drug management.

Environmental

The environmental dimension can be framed as the impact of sport on the natural, physical environment (Smith & Westerbeek, 2007). While the link between environmental responsibility and drug use in sport seems unlikely at first blush, sport does have a responsibility to ensure that drug use has no negative effect on the local and global physical environments.

Sport needs to have policies in place to manage the relationship of sponsors, merchandisers and fans at events when drugs are involved. For example, where sports managers sell access to beverage distributors (e.g. alcohol to fans or sports drinks to participants) it creates the responsibility for cleaning up (e.g. discarded containers) or recycling containers (e.g. encouraging consumers to put containers in recycling bins). The principle of having policies and practices in place to clean up the consequences of drug consumption for the environment extends to other aspects of drug use in sport. For example, the increasing use of injectable drugs to improve aesthetic appeal or strength has seen gymnasiums become a growth area for needle-exchange programmes (Day, Topp, Iversen, & Maher, 2008; Kimergård & McVeigh, 2014). The risks arising from blood-borne viruses from either shared needles or improper disposal of used needles represent a significant threat to non-sport related users of the local physical environment.

Sport's corporate social responsibility to manage drugs in sport

The attempt to manage integrity through managing drugs means sport has to assume responsibility for the breadth of drugs, and the consequences of their consumption. This necessarily takes the notion of 'managing drugs in sport' well beyond anti-doping. For example, agreeing to a sponsorship deal with a local pub may lead to alcohol-related harms among people who would otherwise never interact with sport (e.g. violence or vandalism). As a consequence, sport has a responsibility to society to manage the role drugs play at a number of levels.

The role of anti-doping

It is impossible to discuss drug control-led integrity management in sport without the anti-doping policy being a significant feature. However, it would be incorrect to assume that a discussion about anti-doping is a discussion about drug control in sport. Drug control in sport must consider the role and management of different types of drugs set out in Chapter 2. In part, this book seeks to overcome the assumption that anti-doping is the attempt to manage drugs in sport, and accord it a place as a policy to manage one type of drug consumption.

Having said that, anti-doping plays a dominant role in how all drugs in sport are managed, and was specifically designed to address integrity management concerns. As a result, a large part of the discussion focuses on the implications of the anti-doping policy. In some instances it is the sole focus, simply because anti-doping is the most dominant force for that aspect of management (e.g. governance and risk management). Indeed, a challenge in writing this book was overcoming the tendency to think about drugs in sport purely in terms of anti-doping.

Declaration of position on anti-doping

Writing about anti-doping critically brings with it singular challenges. The management of drugs in sport is an area charged with emotion. For example, the author has been accused of being 'against anti-doping' and 'corrupting sport' for being critical of the management of drugs in sport generally, and anti-doping specifically. Such experience means it is necessary to establish a clear position on the role of drugs in sport for this book.

The author takes the view that drug control is an essential part of managing the integrity of sport. After this point, the decision between anti-doping and any other form of drug control needs to emerge from appropriately critical evaluation of conceptual and empirical evidence. To be clear, the author's interest has been, is and remains in promoting debate around drug control for sport by presenting and critiquing the range of approaches rather than advocating any one approach.

As a result, readers need to be mindful to avoid misconstruing the depth of critiques in relation to anti-doping offered throughout the book as being 'against anti-doping' or 'promoting corruption'. Instead, it is a reflection on the incumbent approach to drug control for sport (anti-doping) also being the focus of most research, and receiving the most critique. The critical review of anti-doping is therefore a function of the depth in thinking on that policy, and the relatively shallow literature on alternatives to which this book seeks to contribute.

Rationale and explanation of the declaration

The reason such a declaration is necessary represents a valuable insight that informs the discussion through the rest of the book. The declaration becomes necessary as a function of both the great myth of sport and the social construction of drug control debates. Coakley (2015) argues that the great sport myth means many see no reason for critical review; that sport is already as it should be. Those critical of the myth are therefore excluded from sport through a range of dissonance-reducing logics. The effect on research critical of drug management in sport is charges of being 'against anti-doping' or seeking to promote inherently 'impure' or 'bad' practices (see Chapter 6).

The social construction of drug debates (Dingelstad, Gosden, Martin, & Vakas, 1996) sees the most powerful interest groups shaping the terms of those debates. Those who oppose the interests of the most powerful groups then have to justify their position based on those terms. In the context of drug control for sport, the terms have been set by the interests of sporting institutions and governments seeking to establish anti-doping as the only possible policy (as argued in Chapters 3 and 4). As a consequence, those who oppose anti-doping have to frame their arguments relative to anti-doping. For example, research published in support of anti-doping rarely has to make claims justifying its position (e.g. anti-doping is self-justifying), whereas research presenting views contrary to anti-doping has to justify its position relative to the anti-doping policy.

The great sport myth and the social construction of drug debates have seen the management of drugs in sport being presented in polarised terms (Mazanov, 2014). Those who support anti-doping typically draw on the 'war on drugs in sport' discourses (Hemphill, 2009; Wagner & Pederson, 2014) to present their policy as self-justifying by defending the virtue of both athletes and sporting institutions from the corrupting taint of drugs (Henne, 2015; Møller, 2014). This discourse demands that opponents of anti-doping be characterised as those who would seek to corrupt both athletes and sporting institutions by making drugs part of sport. By comparison, those who advocate against anti-doping argue that theirs is an enlightened view taking a modern approach to drug control based on evidence drawn from a range of epistemologies (see Dimeo's, 2007, analysis of Hoberman's work). Such discourses characterise advocates of anti-doping as irrationally and unreasonably keeping sport in the dark ages of drug control to benefit sporting institutions at the expense of the integrity of athletes (e.g. Savulescu, 2015). The hyperbole and vitriol arising from the polarised opposition unhelpfully obscures debate that might see progress towards 'second generation' sports drug control policies (Mazanov & Connor, 2010).

How sport manages drugs in sport – structure of the book

The book is divided into three main parts. The first part of the book provides background to the management of drugs in sport. Chapter 2 discusses the role of drugs in sport, presenting a 'sports drug matrix' to demonstrate that the management of drugs in sport necessarily goes well beyond the boundaries of doping. In doing so, an argument is presented that the integrity of sport is best served by addressing the misuse and abuse of drugs generally, rather than managing one type of drug use (doping). Following from this, Chapter 3 provides a historical overview of drug control in sport as a function of drug control in society. The narrative argues that the emergence of anti-doping was a response to the mismanagement of drugs in sport through the late twentieth century. Chapter 4 critiques the anti-doping policy alongside alternative policies defined by a five-stage gradation of drug control from prohibition to permissive.

The second part of the book focuses on the issues that arise from the attempt to implement drug control-led integrity management for sport. Implementation is constructed by considering the implications of drug control for the business of sport (Chapter 5). This is achieved by examining how competing interests in relation to drug control interact, and then looking to the revenue implications of drug control. Chapter 5 structures the remaining discussion of management. Chapter 6 examines the question of managing drugs in sport using business ethics, first by critiquing the values-based approach taken by anti-doping, then offering a CSR-stakeholder values approach and finally providing an overview of how teleological and deontological approaches might inform the management of drugs in sport. Chapter 7 gives an account of the governance arrangements for the anti-doping model as an example of drug control-led integrity management, arguing that success in systemic governance of anti-doping has met with failure in organisational governance. The outcome is that the systemic governance could be adapted to meet any of the policy alternatives offered in Chapter 4. Chapter 8 addresses the risks that arise from the attempt to manage the role of drugs in sport by examining risks that arise from the relationship sport has with different types of drugs (licit, supplements, pharmaceutical and illicit), and how sports organisations are forced to manage the risks associated with anti-doping (e.g. game theory). Given that a key integrity risk for any organisation stems from its personnel, Chapter 9 explores the interaction between standard approaches to CSR and human resource management, arguing for a more sophisticated understanding of their interaction when it comes to managing integrity for sport. The marketing implications of the efforts sport makes in relation to drugs are the final aspect of management practice examined, drawing on the marketing of licit drugs, scandal management, and managing the anti-doping brand (Chapter 10).

The third part looks to broaden the discussion of managing integrity through drug control. Chapter 11 addresses the standing critique that sport acts in the best interests of elite professional male sport at the expense of women, children and non-elite sport. This suggests that the management of drugs in sport could be one way to overcome threats to the integrity of sport arising from the limiting focus on one version of sport. Chapter 12 exploits the existing administrative architecture put in place to give effect to anti-doping to argue for an alternative approach to drug control for sport. Based on harm-minimisation, the alternative approach seeks to preserve the integrity of sport by promoting the integrity of individuals. Chapter 13 draws the discussion together to observe what can be learned from the management of drugs in sport, integrity management in sport, and the management of integrity more broadly.

References

Anderson, L., & Jackson, J. (2013). Competing loyalties in sports medicine: threats to medical professionalism in elite, commercial sport. *International Review for the Sociology of Sport*, *48*(2), 238–256.

Australian University Sport (2009). *Annual Report*. Available at: www.unisport.com.au/inside-aus/governance (accessed 16 November 2015).

Babiak, K. (2010). The role and relevance of corporate social responsibility in sport: A view from the top. *Journal of Management and Organization*, *16*(4), 528–549.

Beddington, J., Cooper, C., Field, J., Goswami, U., Huppert, F., Jenkins, R., *et al.* (2008). The mental wealth of nations. *Nature*, *455*(23), 1057–1060.

Beduschi, G. (2003). Current popular ergogenic aids used in sports: a critical review. *Nutrition and Dietetics*, *60*(2), 104–118.

Bennett, G., Ferreira, M., Lee, J., & Polite, F. (2009). The role of involvement in sports and sport spectatorship in sponsors' brand use: The case of Mountain Dew and action sports sponsorship. *Sport Marketing Quarterly*, *18*(1), 14–24.

Borland, J., & Macdonald, R. (2003). Demand for sport. *Oxford Review of Economic Policy*, *19*(4), 478–502.

Breitbarth, T., Walzel, S., Anagnostopoulos, C., & van Eekeren, F. (2015). Corporate social responsibility and governance in sport: 'Oh, the things you can find, if you don't stay behind!' *Corporate Governance*, *15*(2), 254–273.

Buechel, B., Emrich, E., & Pohlkamp, S. (2014). Nobody's innocent: The role of customers in the doping dilemma. *Journal of Sports Economics*, DOI: 10.1177/1527002514551475

Carroll, A. (1979). A three-dimensional model of corporate performance. *Academy of Management Review*, 4(4), 497–505.

Carstairs, C. (2003). The wide world of doping: Drug scandals, natural bodies, and the business of sports entertainment. *Addiction Research and Theory*, 11(4), 263–281.

Chappelet, J. L. (2011). Towards better Olympic accountability. *Sport in Society*, 14(3), 319–331.

Cisyk, J., & Courty, P. (2015). Do fans care about compliance to doping regulations in sports? The impact of PED suspension in baseball. *Journal of Sports Economics*, DOI: 10.1177/1527002515587441

Coakley, J. (2015). Assessing the sociology of sport: On cultural sensibilities and the great sport myth. *International Review for the Sociology of Sport*, 50(4–5), 402–406.

Connor, J., & Mazanov, J. (2010). The inevitability of scandal: Lessons for sponsors and administrators. *International Journal of Sports Marketing and Sponsorship*, 11(3), 212–220.

Court of Arbitration for Sport (2016). *World Anti-Doping Agency v. Thomas Bellchamber et al., Australian Football League, Australian Sports Anti-Doping Authority*, CAS 2015/A/4059

Crompton, J. (2014). Potential negative outcomes from sponsorship for a sport property. *Managing Leisure*, 19(6), 420–441.

Dahlsrud, A. (2008). How corporate social responsibility is defined: An analysis of 37 definitions. *Corporate Social Responsibility and Environmental Management*, 15(1), 1–13.

Day, C., Topp, L., Iversen, J., & Maher, L. (2008). Blood-borne virus prevalence and risk among steroid injectors: results from the Australian Needle and Syringe Program Survey. *Drug and Alcohol Review*, 27(5), 559–561.

Dimeo, P. (2007). A Critical Assessment of John Hoberman's Histories of Drugs in Sport. *Sport in History*, 27(2), 318–342.

Dingelstad, D., Gosden, R., Martin, B., & Vakas, N. (1996). The social construction of drug debates. *Social Science and Medicine*, 43(12), 1829–1838.

Frenger, M., Emrich, E., & Pitsch, W. (2013). How to produce the belief in clean sports which sells. *Performance Enhancement and Health*, 2(4), 210–215.

Godfrey, P. (2009). Corporate social responsibility in sport: An overview and key issues. *Journal of Sport Management*, 23(6), 698–716.

Hemphill, D. (2009). Performance enhancement and drug control in sport: Ethical considerations. *Sport in Society*, 12(3), 313–326.

Henne, K. (2015). *Testing for Athlete Citizenship*. New Brunswick, NJ: Rutgers University Press.

Kaptein, M. (1999). Integrity management. *European Management Journal*, 17(6), 625–634.

Kimergård, A., & McVeigh, J. (2014). Variability and dilemmas in harm reduction for anabolic steroid users in the UK: A multi-area interview study. *Harm Reduction Journal*, 11(19), 1–13.

Levermore, R. (2013). Viewing CSR through sport from a critical perspective: Failing to address gross corporate misconduct? In J. Paramio-Salcines, K. Babiak, & G. Walters (Eds.), *Routledge Handbook of Sport and Corporate Social Responsibility* (pp. 52–61). Abingdon: Routledge.

Levermore, R., & Moore, N. (2015). The need to apply new theories to 'Sport CSR'. *Corporate Governance, 15*(2), 249–253.

Longbottom, J. (2016). Essendon fined $200,000 over supplements program for breaching workplace safety laws. Available at: www.abc.net.au/news/2016-01-28/essendon-fined-for-failing-to-provide-players-safe-workplace/7120044 (accessed 25 March 2016).

López, B. (2013). Creating fear: The social construction of human growth hormone as a dangerous doping drug. *International Review for the Sociology of Sport, 48*(2), 220–237.

Maennig, W. (2014). Inefficiency of the anti-doping system: Cost reduction proposals. *Substance Use and Misuse, 49*(9), 1201–1205.

Maesschalck, J., & Vanden Auweele, Y. (2010). Integrity management in sport. *Journal of Community and Health Sciences, 5*(1), 1–9.

Marcora, S. (2016). Can doping be a good thing? Using psychoactive drugs to facilitate physical activity behaviour. *Sports Medicine, 46*(1), 1–5.

Mazanov, J. (2014). Drug control in sport: What, how and by whom? In B. Stewart, & M. Burke (Eds.), *Drugs and Sport: Writings from the Edge* (Chapter 2). Melbourne, Australia: Dry Ink Press.

Mazanov, J., & Connor, J. (2010). Rethinking drugs in sport. *International Journal of Sports Policy and Politics, 2*(1), 49–63.

Møller V. (2014). Who guards the guardians? *International Journal of the History of Sport, 31*(8), 934–950.

Møller, V., & Dimeo, P. (2014). Anti-doping – the end of sport. *International Journal of Sport Policy and Politics, 6*(2), 259–272.

Mottram, D. (2015). Drugs and their use in sport. In D. Mottram, & N. Chester (Eds.), *Drugs in Sport (6th Ed)* (pp. 3–20). Oxon: Routledge.

Nicholson, M., & Hoye, R. (2008). Sport and social capital: An introduction. In M. Nicholson, & R. Hoye (Eds.), *Sport and Social Capital* (pp. 1–18). Abingdon: Routledge.

O'Brien, K., & Kypri, K. (2008). Alcohol industry sponsorship and hazardous drinking among sportspeople. *Addiction, 103*(12), 1961–1966.

Orchard, J. W., Steet, E., Massey, A., Dan, S., Gardiner, B., & Ibrahim, A. (2010). Long-term safety of using local anesthetic injections in professional rugby league. *American Journal of Sports Medicine, 38*(11), 2259–2266.

Outram, S., & Stewart, B. (2015). Should nutritional supplements and sports drinks companies sponsor sport? A short review of the ethical concerns. *Journal of Medical Ethics, 41*(6), 447–450.

Paramio-Salcines, J. L. P., Babiak, K., & Walters, G. (Eds.). (2013). *Routledge Handbook of Sport and Corporate Social Responsibility*. Abingdon: Routledge.

Partridge, B., Lucke, J., & Hall, W. (2014). 'If you're healthy you don't need drugs': Public attitudes towards 'brain doping' in the classroom and 'legalised doping' in sport. *Performance Enhancement and Health, 3*(1), 20–25.

Phat, T., Birt, J., Turner, M., & Fenech, J-P (2015). Sporting clubs and scandals – Lessons in governance. *Sport Management Review, 19*(1), 69–80.

Pipe, A., & Ayotte, A. (2002). Nutritional supplements and doping. *Clinical Journal of Sport Medicine, 12*(4), 245–249.

Qureshi, A., Naughton, D., & Petróczi, A. (2014). A systematic review on the herbal extract *Tribulus terrestris* and the roots of its putative aphrodisiac and performance enhancing effect. *Journal of Dietary Supplements, 11*(1), 64–79.

Rowe, N. (2015). Sporting capital: a theoretical and empirical analysis of sport participation determinants and its application to sports development policy and practice. *International Journal of Sport Policy and Politics, 7*(1), 43–61.

Savulescu, J. (2015). Why we should legalise performance-enhancing drugs in sport. In V. Møller, I. Waddington, & J. Hoberman (Eds.), *Routledge Handbook of Drugs and Sport* (pp. 350–362). Abingdon: Routledge.

Sheth, H., & Babiak, K. M. (2010). Beyond the game: Perceptions and practices of corporate social responsibility in the professional sport industry. *Journal of Business Ethics, 91*(3), 433–450.

Smith, E. (2014). Should we fear the role-modelling impact of the anti-doping legislation? *International Journal of Sport Policy and Politics, 6*(2), 273–280.

Smith, A. C., & Westerbeek, H. M. (2007). Sport as a vehicle for deploying corporate social responsibility. *Journal of Corporate Citizenship, 7*(25), 43–54.

Solberg, H., Hanstad, D. V., & Thøring, T. (2010). Doping in elite sport – Do the fans care? Public opinion on the consequences of doping scandals. *International Journal of Sports Marketing and Sponsorship, 11*(3), 185–199.

Stewart, B., & Smith, A. (2014). *Rethinking Drug Use in Sport.* Abingdon: Routledge.

Summers, J., & Johnson, M. (1999). Segmentation of the Australian sport market. In A. Manrai and L. Meadow (Eds.), *Global Perspectives in Marketing for the 21st Century* (pp. 481–486). Heidelberg: Springer International Publishing.

Swann, J. (2015). The history of efforts to regulate dietary supplements in the USA. *Drug Testing and Analysis, 8*(3–4), 271–282.

Treagus, M., Cover, R., & Beasley, C. (2011). *Integrity in Sport.* Canberra: Australian Sports Commission.

Tscholl, P., Junge, A., & Dvorak, J. (2008). The use of medication and nutritional supplements during FIFA World Cups 2002 and 2006. *British Journal of Sports Medicine, 42*(9), 725–730.

Tscholl, P., Alonso, J., Dollé, G., Junge, A., & Dvorak, J. (2010). The use of drugs and nutritional supplements in top-level track and field athletes. *American Journal of Sports Medicine, 38*(1), 133–140.

Tsitsimpikou, C., Tsiokanos, A., Tsarouhas, K., Schamasch, P., Fitch, K., Valasiadis, D., *et al.* (2009). Medication use by athletes at the Athens 2004 Summer Olympic Games. *Clinical Journal of Sport Medicine, 19*(1), 33–38.

Van Reeth, D. (2013). TV demand for the Tour de France: The importance of stage characteristics versus outcome uncertainty, patriotism, and doping. *International Journal of Sport Finance, 8*(1), 39–60.

Wagner, U., & Pederson, K. M. (2014). The IOC and the doping issue – An institutional discursive approach to organisational identity construction. *Sport Management Review, 17*(2), 160–173.

Walker, M., & Parent, M. M. (2010). Toward an integrated framework of corporate social responsibility, responsiveness, and citizenship in sport. *Sport Management Review, 13*(3), 198–213.

Chapter 2

The role of drugs in sport

Drugs have played and continue to play an integral role in modern sport. The aim of this chapter is to establish a two-dimensional framework that enables a more precise discussion of the role of drugs in sport. The first dimension offers a typology to categorise drugs. The second dimension contrasts drug use with misuse and abuse. The implications of this model for drug control-led integrity management in sport are then developed.

The discussion is focused on a general understanding of what drugs are and how they are consumed. It is intended to develop the arguments around how drugs are consumed in sport relative to management rather than give a detailed medical or pharmacological account. Readers interested in such medical accounts may find the latest edition of Mottram and Chester's (2015) *Drugs in Sport* a valuable introduction.

Defining the first dimension: drugs

The word 'drug' is a remarkably ambiguous descriptor that has been applied widely across a range of substances. According to the *Oxford English Dictionary*, a drug was historically used to refer to 'any substance, of animal, vegetable, or mineral origin, used as an ingredient in pharmacy, chemistry, dyeing, or various manufacturing processes'. The definition was refined over time to more specifically refer to 'a natural or synthetic substance used in the prevention or treatment of disease, a medicine' or 'a substance that has a physiological effect on a living organism'.

While the definition suggests that the substance is either natural or synthetic, analysis of how substances influence a living organism mean that the active aspects can be isolated, extracted, purified and refined. In the contemporary context, while a substance may well be natural, by the time it reaches a person in the form of a tablet, powder, suspension or liquid, it has been subjected to a number of manufacturing processes that means it bears little resemblance to its original form. For example, isolated, extracted, purified and refined forms of alcohol bear little resemblance to the original plant.

A common way to understand differences between drugs emerges from their legal status. Prescription drugs are legally controlled, needing formal certification from an accredited medical practitioner to access. Such drugs have been through rigorous testing following the well-established four phase clinical trial method. This evidence is then assessed by relevant health regulators (e.g. the US Food and Drug Administration) before approval for human use. Approval identifies the medical conditions for which the drug is effective, the doses at which it can be safely used and the relative risk of side effects. Over-the-counter drugs have been subjected to clinical trials and demonstrated to be unlikely to have significant health implications (e.g. analgesics such as ibuprofen), but require some instruction in use or to control other implications (e.g. cold tablets containing pseudoephedrine being used to produce methamphetamines). Illicit drugs have usually been adapted from their original therapeutic purpose to emphasise intoxication, sensory or mood effects (e.g. relaxation, euphoria, or visual or auditory hallucinations) that have been deemed harmful to individuals and society, and usually fall under the jurisdiction of criminal rather than health regulation. Licit drugs are widely available, typically through social convention (e.g. caffeine), despite some having clear health implications (e.g. alcohol and nicotine). Supplements are a subset of licit drugs typically touted as refined and purified versions of plants (e.g. St John's Wort) or naturally occurring compounds (e.g. amino acids). Unlike other drugs, the evidence base for their effects is typically drawn from a mix of scientific and non-scientific traditions, and they are generally regarded as having trivial health or criminal implications by regulators.

Defining the second dimension: use, misuse and abuse

Like any technology, use shapes how drugs are understood. Drugs have proven to be both a boon and a bane, with new words being used to more precisely describe the context around how a substance is consumed. That is, new words are introduced that account for the social construction of consumption relative to what is considered acceptable and deviant. For example, when human growth hormone (hGH) is used to overcome the effects of ageing as part of rejuvenation therapy, the normative label 'medicine' conveys the impression of use consistent with intended therapeutic purpose under medical supervision. By contrast, when hGH is used by a young athlete to improve sporting performances, the label 'doping' conveys the impression of dangerously unnecessary and unsupervised abuse well outside the intended therapeutic purpose of the substance (cf. López, 2013).

The characterisation of doping stands in contrast with 'non-medical use' of other therapeutic substances. For example, there has been significant interest in the 'non-medical use of prescription stimulants' among university students to enhance academic performance (e.g. Ford & Ong, 2014; Kerley, Copes, & Griffin, 2015; Ponnet, Wouters, Walrave, Heirman, & van Hal, 2015). That is, university students are taking substances like methylphenidate (drug therapy for attention deficit disorders) or modafinil (drug therapy for narcolepsy) to, presumably, enhance their academic performance (Mazanov, Dunn, Connor, & Fielding, 2013). The descriptor 'non-medical use' suggests that while there has been a transgression in terms of medical supervision and therapeutic need, there is no sense that consumption is likely to be injurious to health. However, when the labels 'neuroenhancement' or 'brain doping' are applied, the connotations change towards becoming socially and medically deviant (Forlini & Racine, 2009).

The difference between drugs and the labels associated with social construction of their use means that understanding the role of drugs in sport, and its management, needs to consider both drugs and the context of their use simultaneously. Drug consumption is typically characterised in terms of use, misuse and abuse.

Use of a drug is established as consumption consistent with recommendations from producers (e.g. pharmaceutical companies) arising from clinical trials, and medical orthodoxy. This can include 'off-label' use, where a drug is re-trialled for a new medical condition or experimental treatment. The decision to use a drug 'off-label' emerges from careful consideration of available evidence about the drug and how it is expected to interact with physiology, and it can require independent approval (e.g. a relevant medical committee) before the drug is used. The key here is that the drug is being consumed based on information derived from rigorous testing or under medical supervision.

The World Health Organisation (2016) defines misuse as consumption of a drug outside legal or medical guidelines, sometimes preferred as a less judgemental term to abuse. However, this definition is unsatisfactory as it fails to provide a meaningful distinction between misuse and abuse. Rather than suggest that misuse is a technical aberration from abuse, a more moderate approach to distinguish misuse from abuse is taken. Misuse is where the drug is being consumed for a purpose other than that for which it has been tested and without reference to medical orthodoxy, or is being used in doses that are inconsistent with producer recommendations. Misuse includes consumption for a desirable side effect of a drug (e.g. weight loss) and people erroneously assuming a substance is going to have any impact on their physical, psychological or spiritual experience. It also includes the failure to understand dose-response relationships; the idea that if one is good, ten must be better. Misuse can also relate to unintentional consumption, such as might occur with an athlete's drink being 'spiked' with flunitrazepam (more commonly known as rohypnol or colloquially as the 'date rape' drug).

Abuse of a drug is systematic consumption well outside intended uses and doses that have a demonstrably negative impact on the health and welfare of an individual and those around them. This includes physical or psychological dependence on the substance (addiction).

Drugs and sport

Mottram (2015) describes four main reasons drugs are of interest to sport:

1   therapeutic use (overcoming a medical condition)
2   performance continuation (treatment of sports injuries)
3   recreational and social (both legal and illegal), and
4   performance enhancement.

Mottram's notion of performance continuation is extended here to include prevention of illness or injury. For example, an athlete may use a drug to boost their immune system in an attempt to prevent minor illnesses such as a cold virus before an important event.

According to Mottram, the role for drugs in sport ranges from specific medical health to helping athletes blow off steam to managing their performance. Importantly, there is a diverse range of both drug-based technologies and ways to consume those drugs under each reason, which have implications relative to use, misuse and abuse. For example, therapeutic use of sleeping tablets can quickly become recreational misuse with significant implications for athletes and their managers (Dunn, 2014; Gearin, 2016). From a managerial point of view, it becomes important to contextualise and understand how different drugs can be used, misused and abused in the sporting context.

The sports drug matrix

Table 2.1 summarises the relationship between the legal status of different substances and their use. Doping is appended to the matrix to enable discussion of what can be learned about that form of drug-taking relative to the others. For example, doping has been used to refer to consumption of licit drugs (e.g. caffeine), supplements (e.g. Jack3d), over-the-counter drugs (e.g. pseudoephedrine), prescription drugs (e.g. anabolic-androgenic steroids) and illicit drugs (e.g. methamphetamine).

Licit drugs

Most licit drugs have penetrated society to the point of ubiquity, noting that some cultural traditions take a different view on some substances (e.g. Christian and Islamic views on alcohol). These drugs are typically used in

Table 2.1 The sports drug matrix

Drug Type	Examples	Use	Misuse	Abuse
Licit	Alcohol Tobacco Caffeine	Social situations Mild effects No short-term health	Excessive use Typically one-off Short-term health	Systematic excess Continuous Health implications
Supplements	Vitamins Protein Creatine	Follow instructions Health promoting Mild or no effect	Ignorance Incorrect dose Short-term health	Excess consumption Erroneous beliefs Licensing
Over-the-counter	Topical steroids Aspirin Decongestants	Follow instructions Minor ailments Medical supervision	Ignorance Incorrect dose Legal highs	Dependence Excess consumption Health implications
Prescription	Beta-blockers Corticosteroids Beta-agonists	Medical supervision Medical conditions Off-label supervised	Unsupervised Legal highs Counter effects	Dependence Excess consumption Health implications
Illicit	Heroin Methamphetamine Ketamine	Functional use Enable work/life Controlled effect	Opportunistic Accidental Incidental	Dependence Excess consumption Health implications
Doping	Pseudoephidrine Anabolic Steroids Erythropoietin	Functional use Enable sport Enhance sport	Unsupervised Accidental Incidental	Dependence Excess consumption Health implications

social situations or as a temporary aid due to their relatively mild effects and short-term effects. For example, coffee can provide a mild stimulating effect without interfering with other activities. Licit drugs can have therapeutic implications, such as certain forms of alcohol in specific amounts being correlated with cardiovascular health (Ronksley, Brien, Turner, Mukamal, & Ghali, 2011).

Misuse of licit substances typically sees the drugs consumed in quantities that exceed general recommendations, making consumers more vulnerable to a range of harms. For example, athletes who consume large quantities of alcohol as part of an isolated event (e.g. a post-tournament celebration) may experience negative effects as a result of that consumption (e.g. unwanted sex). Equally, athletes under pressure in the lead-up to an important event may consume an unusually large number of cigarettes and then revert back to lower use after the event. It is worth noting that misuse of licit substances can lead to significant health consequences, demonstrated by an 18-year-old wrestler dying from a heart attack after consuming a large quantity of anhydrous caffeine (caffeine powder) (Horswill, 2014).

Abuse of licit drugs is where ongoing consumption is systematically excessive. This systematic use typically has short- and long-term health and welfare consequences. For example, an athlete who consumes ten cans of high energy drinks every day is abusing caffeine, with possible consequences including elevated anxiety, inability to sleep, motor control problems (e.g. the jitters) and difficulties with decision making (Harris & Munsell, 2015; Reissig, Strain, & Griffiths, 2009).

Supplements

The reinvigoration of alternative or 'natural' therapies (e.g. naturopathy and herbalism) has seen supplements attract increasing interest from consumers. Supplements are broadly accessible and available for athletes to self-medicate real or perceived conditions. When it comes to performance enhancement, canny marketers advertise supplements as having the same effect on sports performance (e.g. power, endurance or focus) as prohibited drugs (see Chapters 5 and 8). A key part of this strategy is to market supplements as 'natural' alternatives to pharmaceuticals. This claim is problematic from two points of view. The first is, as noted above, the manufacturing processes used to produce many supplements makes them more akin to pharmaceuticals than to their naturally occurring form (e.g. in a flower or herb). The second is that significant variation in supplement production standards leads to contamination with other drugs (Eichner & Tygart, 2015; Maughan, 2013; Petróczi, Taylor, & Naughton, 2011; Pipe & Ayotte, 2002; see Chapter 8). For example, there have been ongoing issues with supplements being contaminated with anabolic steroids (mostly in protein supplements) (e.g. Abbate *et al.*, 2015) and amphetamine analogues (mostly in supplements marketed as 'pre-trainers' that overcome fatigue and improve the quality of training) (Cohen, Travis, & Venhuis, 2014).

With these issues in mind, use of supplements typically follows recommended instructions emerging from a combination of evidence (e.g. medical literature) and experience (e.g. what works in practice). In this regard, athlete use is typically consistent with marketing of supplements as preventatives (e.g. calcium and osteoporosis for female athletes), therapies (e.g. echinacea to reduce the length of a cold during an event) or to enhance performance (e.g. ginkgo biloba for power and endurance).

Misuse can occur on the basis of ignorance, arising from erroneous information or beliefs about effects. For example, athletes may seek to use a supplement on the basis they heard it had an effect without any regard for other evidence. Misuse can also emerge when people use the supplement incorrectly. Misuse of some supplements has no meaningful effect (e.g. multivitamins leading to a change in the colour of urine), but for others it can have profound but hopefully short-term health consequences (e.g. iron overload). A psychological dimension of misuse occurs when athletes begin to believe they are unable to perform without consuming the supplement, even though it has no particular effect on their performance or their health (any change may be the result of placebo effect rather than the supplement) (Beedie & Foad, 2009).

Abuse of supplements arises when they are consumed in large amounts, even when health consequences manifest. For example, athletes continue to consume an iron supplement despite experiencing symptoms of iron overload (such as fatigue). Abuse can also occur where athletes believe the supplements have a compensatory or licensing effect (Chiu, Yang, & Wan, 2011). These effects emerge when athletes adopt a belief that consumption of supplements compensates for the presence of health-diminishing behaviour (e.g. multivitamins and radical weight loss or gain for competition) or gives them 'licence' to abstain from a health-promoting behaviour (e.g. appropriate post-training or post-event recovery periods).

Over-the-counter

Over-the-counter drugs are sold as self-medication for minor ailments. Their status means that use, like supplements, is defined relative to instructions. Over-the-counter drugs can also be considered to be 'used' where a suitably qualified professional (e.g. medical practitioner or pharmacist) advises a deviation from intended use and dose, such as using a drug intended for one purpose to treat another at a significantly higher dose. For example, a medical practitioner may advise paracetamol to be given to athletes prior to competing on a hot day given its capacity to reduce core body temperature (Mauger *et al.*, 2014), rather than as a response to pain (analgesic). Unfortunately, the evidence is less than clear, and may lead athletes to overexert themselves on hot days and place themselves at greater risk of heat strain (licensing effects) (Coombs, Cramer, Ravanelli, Morris, & Jay, 2015).

Taking an over-the-counter drug for an ailment and a dose different to recommendation without suitably qualified advice would constitute misuse, even if that advice is obtained from a source that has been assumed to be reliable. For example, the proliferation of websites that provide information on a range of drugs and their potential to treat a range of conditions means that athletes or support personnel could be confident in the information they are receiving. However, this confidence may be misplaced without clinical judgement taking into account the range of other factors that professionals consider in coming to their advice, such as how the active ingredient works, the other ingredients in the drug and potential contraindications. This judgement may also include whether an over-the-counter preparation contains a prohibited substance (such as topical steroid creams).

Misuse also occurs where an over-the-counter drug is consumed beyond its therapeutic intentions. For example, some over-the-counter drugs can be consumed as 'legal highs'. That is, misuse of the drug leads to some change in visceral or sensory experience, or has intoxicating effects. Misuse of these substances can be appealing to athletes looking for a form of social drug use that minimises the risk of failing a drug test. For example, athletes may consume an over-the-counter drug to 'blow off steam' following competition or as part of a broader social experience (e.g. a party). However, athletes still risk over-the-counter drugs containing prohibited substances. Another form of misuse is when over-the-counter drugs are used as a preventative during competition, such as taking an analgesic before an event to counter anticipated pain. This may license the athlete to ignore pain, making them more vulnerable to injury.

Abuse of over-the-counter drugs follows the pattern of systematic overdose (e.g. if one is good, ten must be better) or dependence that occurs with licit drugs and supplements. Like licit drugs, there are short- and long-term health and welfare consequences of abusing over-the-counter drugs. This may occur where consumption to experience a 'legal high' moves from an occasional misuse to psychological dependence (e.g. superstition) during training, competition and recovery cycles.

Prescription drugs

The conditions for using prescription drugs are very clear. Unlike other drugs, they have specific therapeutic uses so need to be consumed in known doses and in known ways. For example, some drugs need tapering on to get the body used to them before dosing at therapeutic levels and tapering off to avoid withdrawal symptoms. The prescription creates a record that enables monitoring to ensure the drug is having the desired therapeutic effect relative to side effects or contraindications. For instance, the drug may fail to treat the medical condition or lead to side effects that are worse than the condition being treated.

It is possible to use prescription drugs without supervision. Some consumers can become highly educated about prescription drugs such that they are able to use the substance within known safety limits. This may be the case for people who have accurately self-diagnosed and self-medicated conditions, purchasing their drugs through pharmaceutical tourism, intermediaries (e.g. the internet) or the black market (e.g. people with prescriptions selling their drugs, or stolen drugs).

Educated consumers create a grey area between use and misuse. For example, educated consumers may be using a drug or combination of drugs 'off-label' based on personal experience. This approach to drug innovation has something of a tradition in medical sciences, with some famous discoveries being demonstrated by researchers experimenting on themselves (cf. Weisse, 2012). In this instance, educated consumers may be using the substance in the same experimental ways as a medical practitioner might. For example, an educated athlete may find that their endurance improves as a result of treatment for a medical condition. Following rigorous trialling the athlete establishes a dosing regimen that is well within safety limits. This makes it possible for such consumption to be consistent with 'off-label' use rather than being misuse.

Misuse occurs when substances are consumed outside intended therapeutic or justifiable off-label uses. Based on the educated consumer argument, a key to misuse for prescription drugs is that the misuse occurs without insight into how to use the drug. As a result, the 'non-medical use of prescription stimulants' discussed above is a form of misuse under the definitions proposed here. That is, it is more accurate to say 'misuse of prescription stimulants'. Misuse can also occur when countering the effects of another drug. For example, an athlete may look to use a depressant (e.g. barbiturates) to overcome the stimulant effect of their pre-trainer supplement. The 'legal high' phenomenon is also observed for prescription drugs. For example, methylphenidate is sometimes referred to as 'poor man's cocaine' (Forlini & Racine, 2009) and, as noted above, athletes have been known to use sleeping pills as an alternative to other drugs. Finally, misuse emerges when athletes overdose on a prescription drug, perhaps in the belief that taking a higher dose speeds up recovery. A clear misuse of a prescription drug is where that drug is used in the belief that its effect has some impact on sports performance. For example, passing around an albuterol puffer (used to relax airways for asthmatics) before a junior netball game is unlikely to have much effect on health or performance.

Abuse of prescription drugs is a well-known phenomenon. Within the sports drug matrix, abuse is characterised by both dependence and improper doses that lead to significant implications for both health and welfare.

Illicit drugs

It seems a little odd to suggest that illicit drugs could be 'used'. Indeed, some jurisdictions define any consumption of illicit drugs as misuse or abuse. However, drawing on the growing debate around 'functional' use of illicit drugs it is possible to correlate illicit drug use with licit drug use. The operation of the word functional is understood in two ways. The first is that the drug is used to achieve a specific effect, such as increased productivity (Lende, Leonard, Sterk, & Elifson, 2007). The other is that, in contrast with disease models of addiction (where the properties of the drug result in complete loss of control over consumption), self-regulation sees illicit drug use become a functional part of the person's life relative to the health and welfare implications of misuse or abuse (e.g. Zuffa, Meringolo, & Petrini, 2014). That is, the person learns how to control consumption such that it has no socially unacceptable consequences (e.g. missing work or behaving in unacceptable ways). Given that licit drugs can be used for their performance or social effects without interfering with other activities, the same kind of consumption and effects suggest that illicit drugs can also be 'used'.

While use of illicit drugs needs to be argued, misuse of illicit drugs is a more common understanding of consumption. Misuse of illicit drugs is characterised here by non-systematic and less controlled consumption in ways that have implications for health and welfare, such as post-competition celebrations where the drug is consumed opportunistically (e.g. an offer to consume while alcohol-impaired). Misuse also includes accidental consumption, such as marijuana cookies or a cocaine kiss (Duval, 2015). Misuse is distinguished from use and abuse relative to the unknown ingredients, quality or purity of the drugs in the sense that users and abusers are more knowledgeable and concerned about such issues. Inexperienced consumption may see misuse of the illicit drug through consuming the wrong drug (e.g. an ecstasy pill that is actually a cocaine-heroin 'speed ball'), contamination (e.g. quality of chemicals used in production) or at far higher or lower levels of the illicit drug (e.g. heroin cut with icing sugar).

The tragic human cost of illicit drugs is most obvious at the level of abuse. This is the point at which consumption is driven by physical and/or psychological dependence, leading to significant health and welfare implications. Illicit drug abusers no longer exercise control over consumption, often orientating their entire existence towards consumption to the exclusion of other activities. The consequences of abusing illicit drugs stand as the reasons why drug control is necessary both for society and for sport (cf. Mazanov, 2014).

Doping

Surprisingly, the World Anti-Doping Code (the Code) fails to provide a clear definition of doping in terms of drug consumption. For example, under the Code, doping is defined as one of ten anti-doping rule violations (WADA, 2015). This means that doping includes behaviours ranging from testing positive to a prohibited substance to failing to report an anti-doping rule violation. The closest the Code gets to defining doping in terms of consuming drugs is when it relates to a drug on the Prohibited List. Drugs are listed on the Prohibited List when they meet two of three tests; they potentially or actually enhance sporting performance, they potentially or actually pose a health risk to athletes, or they violate the Spirit of Sport statement (see Chapter 4). As a result, the range of drugs considered to be 'doping' extends from illicit drugs (marijuana) to over-the-counter drugs (e.g. diuretics used to 'mask' other drug use) to prescription drugs (anabolic steroids). For the purposes of discussion here, a colloquial understanding of doping is applied – doping refers to drugs consumed for the purposes of enhancing sporting performance.

Drugs consumed for the purposes of enhancing sporting performance are drawn from across the spectrum of licit drugs, supplements, over-the-counter drugs, prescription drugs and illicit drugs. This means that characterising their use, misuse and abuse also draws on those arguments.

If the purpose of an athlete is to produce sporting performances, using drugs that enable or enhance sporting performances is functional to the athlete's social context (Petróczi & Aidman, 2008). Athletes are able to 'use' doping when that drug is absent from the Prohibited List. This means that drugs which clearly enhance sporting performance, like caffeine, can be used by athletes. Indeed, the absence of caffeine from the Prohibited List has seen the development of a precise science to maximise the stimulant effects of caffeine for sport (Burke, Desbrow, & Spriet, 2013). For example, athletes can be assessed for how caffeine changes their sports performances and given a dosage timed to have an impact at various points in an event. The point here is that unlike the social construction of doping as a dangerously unsupervised and unnecessary consumption, doping can be a legitimate and important part of sport.

Misuse is both straightforward and challenging for how doping might be understood. Among the straightforward issues, misuse of doping occurs when consumption is inconsistent with manufacturer instructions or medical orthodoxy. For example, an athlete taking too much caffeine at the wrong times constitutes misuse of doping. Another misuse of doping is assuming that a substance that enhances one aspect of sports performance is going to positively impact all sports performance. For example, an athlete may erroneously think that taking methylphenidate is going to build muscle mass. A challenging issue is the idea that giving an athlete a drug that enhances sporting performance without their knowledge constitutes misuse. To be clear, this represents misuse by the athlete. Those administering the drugs without the athlete's knowledge are committing a serious harm; thus, German Democratic Republic athletes were misusing doping while those administering the drugs and managing the programme were engaged in an entirely different set of behaviours.

Abuse of doping occurs when consumption crosses the threshold of impugning athlete health and welfare. While the physiological consequences of anabolic steroid abuse are well known, the identification of Anabolic Steroid Dependence Disorder (Kanayama, Brower, Wood, Hudson, & Pope, 2009) as a serious substance dependence disorder took much longer to identify, with characteristics similar to both opioid (e.g. withdrawal and continued use despite adverse effects) and nicotine dependence (e.g. no immediate compromise on performance or intoxicating effects).

Implications of the sports drug matrix for managing drugs in sport

The key implication of the sports drug matrix is that sport needs to be explicitly concerned with managing the full range of drugs across the different ways they can be used (cf. Stewart & Smith, 2014). The introduction of the World Anti-Doping Code has seen the focus of drug management for sport concentrate on doping, which represents only one subset of drugs that have implications for sport. For example, managing drugs in sport needs to be as concerned with alcohol abuse, misuse of iron supplements, abuse of sleeping tablets or heroin addiction as it is with the role of erythropoietin.

The sports drug matrix puts in place an argument that the integrity of sport is contingent upon addressing the use, misuse and abuse of drugs generally rather than the misuse or abuse of doping (the example of caffeine demonstrating that use of drugs that enhance performance is acceptable). The focus on doping has distracted debate around drug management for sport. This is perhaps understandable as doping has been constructed as having the most significant impact on the integrity of sport in terms of policy discourses (Wagner & Pedersen, 2014), anxiety about its impact on revenues (Carstairs, 2003; see Chapter 5) and the architecture of international sports management (e.g. anti-doping compliance to access Olympic events). However, in doing so, sports managers appear to have missed important implications about drug control that impact on the integrity of sport, such as managing so-called 'negative doping', where athletes are given drugs to impair performance (Lippi, Sanchis-Gomar, & Banfi, 2012; see Chapter 5). The sports drug matrix suggests that the primary focus of drug control-led integrity management for sport should be to put drugs first and sport second.

The focus on managing doping rather than drugs in sport has had necessary resource implications, with the international effort to establish and implement the anti-doping policy robbing other forms of drug control of resources. Evidence of this can be seen in the adaptation of anti-doping to illicit drug management (e.g. ASC, 2010). This sort of adaptation is a rational response in a resource constrained environment (see Chapter 7). It is perhaps time for managers to refocus resources on achieving effective management of drug use, misuse and abuse in sport. For example, sports managers could look to reinvest cost savings achieved by minimising administrative anti-doping compliance activities into developing programme level understanding of drug use, misuse and abuse (see Chapter 9).

Refocusing on use, misuse and abuse may see doping reabsorbed into other drugs. The idea that a drug has implications for performance enhancement in sport could be reconstructed as use. Caffeine was chosen to make the point about doping use as an uncontroversial and socially acceptable example. However, the point about caffeine generalises to other drugs. That is, developing the science of drug consumption for sport may see more doping classified as 'off-label' use. For example, anabolic-androgenic steroids have had a long history in sports medicine that demonstrates both effect and safety implications in the sporting context (Harmer, 2010). As a result, medically supervised consumption of anabolic steroids is well within medical orthodoxy. This line of argument extends to newer drugs such as erythropoietin, where clinical trials would be needed to demonstrate both the effect and its safety implications for sport. It is difficult to see such trials going ahead in the context of the anti-doping policy. However, under the sports drug matrix, the conclusion of clinical trials around 'off-label' use could see doping become classified as over-the-counter or prescription drugs.

Absorbing doping into other classifications in the sports drug matrix also has the benefit of more clearly addressing the role of illicit drugs in sport. The inclusion of illicit drugs such as marijuana on the Prohibited List has led to significant debate about whether the anti-doping policy is about the integrity of sport or the control and exploitation of athletes (Waddington, Christiansen, Gleaves, Hoberman, & Møller, 2013).

In terms of integrity management, the focus on doping has created a moral panic about one specific form of drug use (Coomber, 2014; Crichter, 2014; Goode, 2015; McDermott, 2016). Sport has bet its integrity on responding to doping when it could gain more in terms of integrity management by addressing drug consumption more broadly. The starting point for a shift in the reciprocal expectations of producers and consumers is to acknowledge that drugs have an important role in sport whether supporting the immune system, assisting recovery or promoting physical literacy. Absorbing doping into existing forms of drug use, misuse and abuse allows the moral panic to dissipate and for sport to focus on the critical issue of drug abuse in sport, whether alcohol, iron supplements, cough mixtures, sleeping tablets, amphetamines or anabolic steroids.

References

Abbate, V., Kicman, A. T., Evans-Brown, M., McVeigh, J., Cowan, D. A., Wilson, C. *et al.* (2015). Anabolic steroids detected in bodybuilding dietary supplements – A significant risk factor to public health. *Drug Testing and Analysis, 7*(7), 609–618.

ASC (2010). *Illicit Drugs in Sport Policy.* Canberra: Australian Sports Commission. Available at www.clearinghouseforsport.gov.au/__data/assets/pdf_file/0007/395062/ASC-illicit-drugs-policy-2010-2014-watermarked.pdf (accessed 9 February 2016).

Beedie, C. J., & Foad, A. J. (2009). The placebo effect in sports performance. *Sports Medicine, 39*(4), 313–329.

Burke, L., Desbrow, B., & Spriet, L. (2013). *Caffeine for Sports Performance.* Champaign, IL: Human Kinetics.

Carstairs, C. (2003). The wide world of doping: Drug scandals, natural bodies, and the business of sports entertainment. *Addiction Research and Theory, 11*(4), 263–281.

Chiu, W. B., Yang, C. C., & Wan, C. S. (2011). Ironic effects of dietary supplementation: Illusory invulnerability created by taking dietary supplements licenses health risk behaviours. *Psychological Science, 22*(8), 1081–1086.

Cohen, P. A., Travis, J. C., & Venhuis, B. J. (2014). A methamphetamine analog (N,alpha-diethyl-phenylethylamine) identified in a mainstream supplement. *Drug Testing and Analysis, 6*(7–8), 805–807.

Coomber, C. (2014). How social fear of drugs in the non-sporting world creates a framework for doping policy in the sporting world. *International Journal of Sport Policy and Politics, 6*(2), 171–193.

Coombs, G. B., Cramer, M. N., Ravanelli, N. M., Morris, N. B., & Jay, O. (2015). Acute acetaminophen ingestion does not alter core temperature or sweating during exercise in hot-humid conditions. *Scandinavian Journal of Science and Medicine in Sports, 25*(S1), 96–103.

Crichter, C. (2014). New perspectives on anti-doping policy: From moral panic to moral regulation. *International Journal of Sport Policy and Politics, 6*(2), 153–159.

Dunn, M. (2014). The importance of understanding motives for prescription substance use and misuse in sport. *Performance Enhancement and Health, 3*(2), 102–104.

Duval, A. (2015). Cocaine, doping and the Court of Arbitration for Sport. *The International Sports Law Journal, 15*(1–2), 55–63.

Eichner, A., & Tygart, T. (2015). Adulterated dietary supplements threaten the health and sporting career of up-and-coming young athletes. *Drug Testing and Analysis*, 8(3–4), 304–306.

Ford, J. A., & Ong, J. (2014). Non-medical use of prescription stimulants for academic purposes among college students: a test of social learning theory. *Drug and Alcohol Dependence*, 144(November 1), 279–282.

Forlini, C., & Racine, E. (2009). Disagreements with implications: Diverging discourses on the ethics of non-medical use of methylphenidate for performance enhancement. *BMC Medical Ethics*, 10(1).

Gearin, M. (2016). Swimming Australia boss criticises handling of London 2012 Olympics scandals ahead of Rio 2016. Available at: www.abc.net.au/news/2016-02-07/swimming-australia-boss-criticises-london-2012-scandals/7147114 (accessed 9 February 2016).

Goode, E. (2015). Is concern about sports doping a moral panic? In V. Møller, I. Waddington, & J. Hoberman (Eds.), *Routledge Handbook of Drugs and Sport* (pp. 31–40). Abingdon: Routledge.

Harmer, P. A. (2010). Anabolic-androgenic steroid use among young male and female athletes: Is the game to blame? *British Journal of Sports Medicine*, 44(1), 26–31.

Harris, J. L., & Munsell, C. R. (2015). Energy drinks and adolescents: What's the harm? *Nutrition Reviews*, 73(4), 247–257.

Horswill, I. (2014). Eighteen-year-old Logan Stiner dies from taking too much caffeine powder. Available at: www.news.com.au/lifestyle/health/eighteenyearold-logan-stiner-dies-from-taking-too-much-caffeine-powder/news-story/ee98547d0d285905264d8c108be8fb97 (accessed 9 February 2016).

Kanayama, G., Brower, K. J., Wood, R. I., Hudson, J. I., & Pope, H. G. (2009). Anabolic-androgenic steroid dependence: An emerging disorder. *Addiction*, 104(12), 1966–1974.

Kerley, K. R., Copes, H., & Griffin, O. H. (2015). Middle-class motives for non-medical prescription stimulant use among college students. *Deviant Behavior*, 36(7), 589–603.

Lende, D. H., Leonard, T., Sterk, C. E., & Elifson, K. (2007). Functional methamphetamine use: The insider's perspective. *Addiction Research and Theory*, 15(5), 465–477.

Lippi, G., Sanchis-Gomar, F., & Banfi, G. (2012). Anti-'negative-doping' testing: a new perspective in anti-doping research? *European Journal of Applied Physiology*, 112(6), 2383–2384.

López, B. (2013). Creating fear: The social construction of human growth hormone as a dangerous doping drug. *International Review for the Sociology of Sport*, 48(2), 220–237.

Mauger, A. R., Taylor, L., Harding, C., Wright, B., Foster, J., & Castle, P. C. (2014). Acute acetaminophen (paracetamol) ingestion improves time to exhaustion during exercise in the heat. *Experimental Physiology*, 99(1), 164–171.

Maughan, R. (2013). Quality assurance issues in the use of dietary supplements, with special reference to protein supplements. *Journal of Nutrition*, 143(11), 1843S–1847S.

Mazanov, J. (2014). Drug control in sport: Who and how. In B. Stewart & M. Burke (Eds.), *Drugs and Sport: Writings from the Edge* (pp. 33–71). Melbourne: Dry Ink Press.

Mazanov, J., Dunn, M., Connor, J., & Fielding, M. L. (2013). Substance use to enhance academic performance among Australian university students. *Performance Enhancement and Health*, 2(3), 110–118.

McDermott, V. (2016). *The War on Drugs in Sport: Moral Panics and Organizational Legitimacy*. Abingdon: Routledge.

Mottram, D. (2015). Drugs and their use in sport. In D. Mottram & N. Chester (Eds.), *Drugs in Sport (6th Ed)* (pp. 3–20). Abingdon: Routledge.

Mottram, D., & Chester, N. (Eds.). (2015). *Drugs in Sport (6th Ed.)*. Abingdon: Routledge.

Petróczi, A., & Aidman, E. (2008). Psychological drivers of doping: The life-cycle model of performance enhancement. *Substances Abuse Treatment, Prevention and Policy*, 3(7).

Petróczi, A., Taylor, G., & Naughton, D. (2011). Mission impossible? Regulatory and enforcement issues to ensure safety of dietary supplements. *Food and Chemical Toxicology*, 49(2), 393–402.

Pipe, A., & Ayotte, C. (2002). Nutritional supplements and doping. *Clinical Journal of Sport Medicine*, 12(4), 245–249.

Ponnet, K., Wouters, E, Walrave, E., Heirman, W., & van Hal, G. (2015). Predicting students' intention to use stimulants for academic performance enhancement. *Substance Use and Misuse*, 50(3), 275–282.

Reissig, C. J., Strain, E. C., & Griffiths, R. R. (2009). Caffeinated energy drinks – a growing problem. *Drug and Alcohol Dependence*, 99(1), 1–10.

Ronksley, P. E., Brien, S. E., Turner, B. J., Mukamal, K. J., & Ghali, W. A. (2011). Association of alcohol consumption with selected cardiovascular disease outcomes: A systematic review and meta-analysis. *British Medical Journal*, 342(d671).

Stewart, B., & Smith, A. (2014). *Rethinking Drug Use in Sport*. Abingdon: Routledge.

WADA (2015). *World Anti-Doping Code*. Montreal: World Anti-Doping Agency.

Waddington, I., Christiansen, A. V., Gleaves, J., Hoberman, J., & Møller, V. (2013). Recreational drug use and sport: Time for a WADA rethink? *Performance Enhancement and Health*, 2(2), 41–47.

Wagner, U., & Pedersen, K. M. (2014). The IOC and the doping issue – An institutional discursive approach to organizational identity construction. *Sport Management Review*, 17(2), 160–173.

Weisse, A. B. (2012). Self-experimentation and its role in medical research. *Texas Heart Institute Journal*, 39(1), 51–54.

World Health Organisation (2016). Lexicon of alcohol and drug terms. Available at: www.who.int/substance_abuse/terminology/who_lexicon/en/ (accessed 9 February 2016).

Zuffa, G., Meringolo, P., & Petrini, F. (2014). Cocaine users and self-regulation mechanisms. *Drugs and Alcohol Today*, 14(4), 194–206.

Chapter 3

The evolution of drug control for sport

The evolution of drug control for sport is contextualised next to drug control in broader society. This approach assumes a hierarchy where drug control for sport is a subset of the broader effort to manage drugs. That is, the issue is fundamentally one of drug control first and sport second, suggesting that sports managers could learn a great deal about drug control by extrapolating the lessons learned from other market sectors (e.g. the government sector). Instead, the development of drug control unique to sport saw twentieth-century sports managers engaging in symbolic actions creating opportunities for other stakeholders to seize the initiative. Sports managers regained some of the initiative in the early twenty-first century with the anti-doping policy. It remains to be seen whether sports managers have learned the lessons of the past relative to emerging questions of drug control for sport.

From ancient times to the Renaissance

The foundations of modern drug control began with ancient social conventions around alcohol consumption. Alcohol (in the form of grape wine) appears to have emerged from China around 7000–6600 BCE before spreading to the rest of the world (Chrzan, 2013). While alcohol was noted for its intoxicating and medicinal effects, it was typically diluted to make water potable by killing bacteria. Like other intoxicating substances (such as opium), more concentrated or pure forms were reserved for medical practice, the wealthy or for significant occasions (e.g. harvest festivals or the Eucharist).

The foundations of modern drug control in sport stem from the Greek merging of religion and sport to create the ancient Olympics. As a religious festival to honour Zeus, athletes had to swear they had committed no sin or perjury, and that they had abided by the regulations for training for the previous ten months (Crowther, 1996). Competitors at the ancient Olympics often used special diets (e.g. eating specific animal organs) or drank elixirs (e.g. combinations of herbs with stimulant effects) as an integral part of both preparation and competition (Crowther, 2002; Yesalis & Bahrke, 2002). All athletes potentially had access to some special diet or potion they felt would influence sports performances. It therefore seems unlikely that the managers of the ancient Olympics, the *Hellanodikai*, were particularly concerned about such issues. Indeed, any concerns about diets or elixirs would probably have been treated as a trivial distraction next to the rampant cheating and corruption in the ancient Olympics (Kyle, 2015). (Notably, evidence is beginning to suggest that the demise of the ancient Olympics was a result of centralised administration and financial crises, rather than cheating and corruption; Remijsen, 2015.) Of interest to the evolution of drug control for sport is the idea that athletes must be held accountable to a standard and that sporting transgressions were divinely offensive. That is, the integrity of sport correlates with divinity rather than humanity (cf. Ritchie, 2014).

Religion continued to play a dominant role in drug control in the Ancient and Middle Ages and the Renaissance. For example, the use of alcohol was regulated in different ways according to different religions, from drunken Dionysian orgies to the prohibition of alcohol consumption in Islam. Tobacco was generally used as part of important spiritual ceremonies by Native North American peoples, including the exhaled tobacco smoke transporting thoughts or prayers to heaven (Winter, 2000). Following the introduction of tobacco to Europe, religion continued to exert significant influence around tobacco control. The seventeenth century saw Pope Urban VIII threaten to excommunicate snuff users, later followed by a series of Papal Bulls controlling tobacco use by both priests and congregation (Buescher, 2012; Goodman, 2005).

Pre-industrial drug control

The European colonisation of the Americas saw the emergence of powerful tobacco companies. Increasing popularity in Europe meant the export of tobacco became a primary source of revenue for new colonies in North America through the seventeenth and eighteenth centuries. Governments across the world adopted different control measures, including execution (China, Russia and Turkey) and prohibition (Switzerland) (Burns, 2009). These control measures folded in the face of normalisation of smoking (e.g. monarchs who enjoyed tobacco repealing controls) and the tax revenues that could be collected from the tobacco trade. Colonial governments built their wealth from revenues (e.g. export duties) collected in connection with the tobacco economy (Rabushka, 2010), which included the importation of manufactured goods from Europe and slavery. Importantly, the wealth underpinning the tobacco companies saw those who owned them secure and grow their political power base, with significant roles in nation building both in America (e.g. Breen, 2009) and the British Empire (e.g. Devine, 1976).

While European colonialists were learning the lessons of tobacco control, opium control brought with it a different set of lessons. China first listed opium as a taxable commodity in CE 1589 (Yangwen, 2005) which regulated the drug for a range of performance enhancing, medicinal and recreational uses. The impact of opium on the Emperor's administrators saw the first ban for all but small medicinal doses in CE 1729, and complete prohibition from CE 1799 (Yangwen, 2005). The British used the prohibition to corner the opium smuggling market into China by exploiting European access to China through India. While the British Empire became increasingly wealthy from opium, China suffered the public crisis of widespread opium addiction (Hanes & Sanello, 2004). The inevitably strong response from the Chinese government to rescue its people from the epidemic led to the First and Second Opium Wars of the nineteenth century, where China was forced to legalise opium in the context of inequitable terms of trade.

Pre-industrial era drug control was therefore driven by trade. From the point of view of consumers, producers and governments, tobacco control was a question of wealth transfer at the expense of the human interests of those forced to be their slaves. By contrast, the opium trade demonstrated the shortcomings of drug control through taxation, with the crippling of China through nationwide drug misuse and abuse setting the scene for future governmental drug control.

The emergence of modern sport

The emergence of modern sport in the late nineteenth and early twentieth centuries was shaped by the colonial legacy of the British Empire, where sport was used to civilise those deemed in need of moral improvement. This moralising of sport occurred through the lens of a particular interpretation of Protestantism known as 'muscular Christianity' (Hall, 1994; MacAloon, 2013; Putney, 2001), which inculcated concepts like naturalness, fairness and the Protestant work ethic into sport. These ideas drew on romanticised interpretations about the integrity of ancient Olympians demonstrating faith through sport (Ritchie, 2014). This contributed to the creation of a mythology that sport was an intrinsically virtuous activity, such that to transgress against sport was to transgress against the divine. The ideas used to mythologise sport as a virtuous activity represent the foundation to the romanticised values transmitted through successive models of sports management that distinguish drug control for sport from attempts to control drugs in other social contexts (see Chapters 4 and 6).

The late nineteenth century saw modern sport emerge as a natural laboratory to explore the expanding pharmacopoeia (Dimeo, 2007). Scientists used endurance events like cycling and the marathon to test the effect of various substances or combinations of substances on the human organism (Hoberman, 1992). The rise of sports consumerism and the attendant interest in professional sport saw drug consumption emerge as an integral part of sporting practice. For example, participation in extreme sporting spectacles such as the Tour de France saw riders use various combinations of drugs to remain internally competitive and keep the sport externally competitive by delivering the sensations necessary to attract and retain consumer interest (Hoberman, 1992), and this has remained a feature of professional cycling throughout its history (Brewer, 2002).

Industrialisation

By the nineteenth century, industrialisation and the explosion in the natural sciences had a significant impact on drug control. The distillation of alcohol was transformed by industrialisation, enabling purer forms of alcohol to become cheaper and more accessible. In turn, increased alcohol consumption increased alcohol-based tax revenues to governments. However, the crisis of nationwide opium addiction in China appeared to repeat as the West struggled to come to terms with the implications of widespread misuse and abuse of concentrated alcohol (e.g. spirits). As the social impacts of alcohol misuse and abuse manifested, grass-roots movements aimed at establishing alcohol control in the social rather than economic interest were championed by predominantly Protestant religious groups (Hamm, 1995). The Temperance Movement of the United States successfully lobbied for the prohibition of alcohol from 1920 to 1933 (Hall, 2010). The initial decline in alcohol consumption disappeared by 1921. Instead of controlling alcohol misuse and abuse, prohibition appears to have caused governments to forgo tax revenue while increasing the costs of law enforcement to deal with alcohol-related organised crime (black markets, gangsterism and police corruption).

Even though the Great Depression makes it difficult to attribute causality for the failure of prohibition, the lessons from the alcohol prohibition policy experiment remain important to modern drug control (Levine & Reinarman, 1991). Among the many lessons, three are particularly relevant to drug control for sport. The first was that governments needed to do more than collect taxes in the face of widespread drug misuse and abuse. The second was that prohibition can be an expensive and ineffective form of drug control. The third was that consumers and governments were willing to impose external regulation if drug producers failed to act in the public interest.

While the alcohol industry experienced external regulation, tobacco companies were coming to the full height of their industrialised powers, having seen off several challenges to regulate production and consumption in the United States (Lesch & Middendorf-Brand, 1997). Industrial scale production brought with it sufficient revenues to justify extraordinary marketing budgets. Part of these marketing budgets was used to give free cigarettes to soldiers through the First World War, leading to a remarkable increase in the consumer base after the war (Brandt, 2007). These budgets were also used to exploit new technologies emerging from the industrial era, such as radio and cinema advertising (e.g. Lum, Polansky, Jackler, & Glantz, 2008). With tobacco consumption normalised as an acceptable and at times expected social behaviour in the Industrialised West, advertising sought to achieve brand loyalty through consumers linking personal identity with a particular product. Alongside their extraordinary marketing budgets, tobacco companies used their position in the market (e.g. tax receipts, employment and lobbying) to exercise extraordinary political power that ensured the interests of tobacco companies were at the centre of government control of their industry.

As industrialisation increased the supply of existing drugs, the natural sciences expanded the pharmacopoeia with new agents isolated, refined and machine produced – such as new forms of opium (e.g. laudanum and morphine) and cocaine (e.g. coca cola syrup). The effects of the Opium Wars (both revenue and public health) saw governments take an interest in controlling access to new pharmaceuticals, and especially narcotics derived from opium and cocaine. In the United States, the Harrison Narcotics Tax Act of 1914 was introduced to control the buying and selling of both drugs. The United Kingdom began the transition towards tighter control with the 1920 Dangerous Drugs Act seeing opium-related products moved from being an over-the-counter to a prescription substance (Anderson & Berridge, 2000) Importantly, these drugs were controlled separately to the alcohol and tobacco industries, beginning the separation of licit from other drugs (see Chapter 2).

The emergence of drug control for sport

It is within the context of an expanding pharmacopoeia, industrialisation, increasing government regulation and moralising of drug control that modern sport and the resurrected Olympics began to consider the role and control of drugs in sport. The early twentieth century debate around drug control in sporting contexts appears to have been subsumed as part of the broader debate about amateurism – characterised as the 'clean amateurs' and the 'doped professionals' (Gleaves, 2011; Gleaves & Llewellyn, 2014). In essence, the debate pitched the intrinsic virtue of participation against those who would seek extrinsic benefit by making their living from sport. The view that consuming substances to enhance performance diminishes the intrinsic (divine) virtue of amateurism, and later, sport more generally, has echoed throughout the history of drug management in sport.

The International Amateur Athletic Federation began to include bans for doping as early as 1928, ostensibly to protect amateurs at the expense of professionals (Gleaves, 2011). By 1938 the Olympic movement had released its first statement against the notion of 'doping' (Gleaves & Llewellyn, 2014). At this point sports managers were beginning to construct drugs as something that threatened the great sporting myth (Ritchie, 2014); the principle of amateurism being used as a representation or summary of what made sport intrinsically valuable. In doing so, while drug management was described using the catch-all idea that it was responding to 'doping', it actually addressed the use of a range of licit, over-the-counter, prescription and illicit drugs in sport. Unlike the omnipotent and omniscient divine guardian of the ancient Olympics, the modern Olympics had no reliable test for whether an athlete had 'doped'. As a result, the early debate around the role of performance enhancing drugs in sport was largely ideological rather than practical. Importantly, it was this debate that began to shape the rules- and values-based expectations that would shape drug control policy for sport (Ritchie, 2014).

Post-war drug control: the war on drugs

While the intervention of the Second World War saw a pause in progress on the debate around drug control for sport, the debate around drug control in society intensified. The mid-twentieth century saw a second surge in the pharmacopoeia following advances in the physical sciences made as a result of the war. For example, the penetration of anabolic-androgenic steroids and amphetamines into society and sport has its roots in the Second World War (Yesalis & Bahrke, 2002). The competition for market share among pharmaceutical companies intensified after the war, with research driving innovation in drug technology at a breathtaking rate. The primary target for these markets was over-the-counter and prescription drugs which saw an increasing acceptance of medicating people in response to social rather than medical concerns (e.g. using drugs to medicate 'happiness'; Herzberg, 2009).

The unprecedented level of innovation in drug technologies saw new types of synthetic drugs emerge that had no apparent therapeutic implications, such as the psychotropic drug lysergic acid diethylamide, or LSD. Consumption of drugs such as marijuana or LSD began to emerge as a central part of practice among post-war counter cultures (Lee, 2012; Lee & Shlain, 1985). The proliferation and normalisation of drug use among these counter cultures saw governments strengthen regulation and criminalisation, creating the modern concept of an 'illicit drug' (see Chapter 2). The religious moralising of drug consumption arising from the Papal Bulls on tobacco and focused by the Temperance Movement re-emerged with the demonisation of illicit drugs (cf. Coomber, 2014). With the lessons of the Opium Wars and alcoholism apparent, evidence from public health advocates emerged demonstrating the impact of illicit drug misuse and abuse in the late twentieth century across a range of illicit substances, from marijuana to heroin to cocaine to amphetamines. Such evidence saw drug control become far more formalised, attracting increasing regulation through the late twentieth century.

By the 1970s, the declaration of the prohibitionist 'war on drugs' in the United States (US) drew together the interests in controlling tax revenue, the religious moralising discourses and public health arguments. Drugs such as LSD were criminalised, despite experimentation by both the United Kingdom and United States governments (Bergen-Cico, 2012). Prohibition quickly translated to the rest of the world through the United Nations, where the United States exploited its disproportionate financial support by allegedly threatening to withdraw drug control funding if its preferred prohibitionist approach received insufficient international support (Bewley-Taylor, 2005). As a result, United Nations drug control treaties compelled international policy harmonisation based on the prohibitionist approach. This represents the point at which modern regulation of licit, over-the-counter, prescription and illicit drugs came into effect.

The war on drugs in sport begins

The emergence of sports science in the post-Second World War era saw a return to interest in the adaptation of drugs for sporting purposes, in particular anabolic steroids and amphetamines (Dimeo, 2007). Like the late nineteenth century, sport was once again a natural laboratory for testing the effects of new substances on human performance. As the sophistication and potency of the drugs improved, so too did the consequences of their naive misuse and abuse (noting that little was known about these new substances at the time); this is typified by the death of Knud Jensen (Mazanov & McDermott, 2009) and the misattribution of Tommy Simpson's death to amphetamines (López, 2014). The gravity of the consequences for drug misuse and abuse forced the management of drugs in sport to evolve from a conceptual to a practical debate (Beamish & Ritchie, 2004). By the 1960s the management of drugs in sport augmented the ideological arguments seen prior to the Second World War with the stark pragmatism of preventing athlete deaths arising from misuse or abuse.

Following the lead of the war on drugs, the scene was set for the formalisation of drug control in sport. Three policy experiments to manage drugs in sport began. The first experiment drew on professional sport's protection of commercial interests. The Cold War provided the backdrop for the development of two very different policies aiming to manage drugs in amateur sport, divided by the Iron Curtain.

Professional sport

The post-war years retained the historically sharp distinction between amateur and professional sport. As a result, drug control in professional sport developed largely independently of amateur sport. The distinction between amateur and professional sports drug control effectively disappeared by the early twenty-first century, with non-Olympic professional sport being forced to adopt the Olympic approach to drug control as a function of the global Olympic hegemony (Stewart, Adair, & Smith, 2011; Wagner, 2011).

While professional and amateur sport were still distinct, and with the approaching war on drugs, professional sports in the United States (the National Football League, Major League Baseball and the National Basketball Association) established drug control for players' use of licit, prescription and illicit substances based on their commercial implications. Sports managers were keen to avoid drug scandals that appeared to spook consumers and sponsors, diminishing returns on investment (Voy, 1991). At the same time sports managers were keen to exploit new drug technologies that helped players produce sporting spectacles, such as drugs to help keyed up athletes sleep or recover more quickly from injuries. This led to the development of a negotiated drug control system that set up clauses in employment contracts and established a list of controlled substances, testing regimes and consequences for testing positive to a controlled substance (e.g. at what point a contract could be terminated) (Masteralexis, 2006). Importantly, power inequities appear to have shaped drug control for professional sport in favour of leagues, team owners and sports managers (Bennett, 2013). This was the dominant approach to drug control for professional sport for the remainder of the twentieth century.

Amateur sport

In contrast to professional sport, drug control for amateur sport was being shaped by the changing status of the Olympics. On the one hand, the debate around amateurism intensified with the increasing interest in professional rather than Olympic sport. On the other hand, pre-war politicisation of the Olympics was exacerbated by the Cold War. In the absence of direct conflict between the West and Soviet Bloc countries, sport became a battleground to test the ideological superiority of democratic capitalism and dictatorial communism (Hunt, 2007; Mazanov & McDermott, 2009). This saw a confused and sometimes contradicting set of discourses emerge around drugs in sport (Wagner & Pedersen, 2014). Increasing concerns about the health implications of drug use in sport were integrated with political discourses serving the Cold War, which were simultaneously adapted and radicalised to raise a new ethics of drugs in sport (Ritchie,

2014). As a consequence, some leading actors labelled drug consuming athletes 'evil' and 'morally dulled' (Porritt, 1965, pp. 47–49). These discourses became the ideological foundation for the future anti-doping policy.

The Cold War saw very different approaches to drug control on either side of the Iron Curtain. Soviet Bloc countries resourced sophisticated networks to control athlete drug use, misuse and abuse, the most prominent examples of which were state-sponsored doping in the German Democratic Republic (Ungerleider, 2001) and the People's Republic of China (Leonard, 2001). While state-sponsored systems led to egregious exploitation and abuses of young men and women for the sake of political posturing, the evidence suggests that there were very strict controls around drug administration that made some effort to protect athlete health (Hunt, Dimeo, Hemme, & Mueller, 2014). The effectiveness of Soviet sports drug management regimes saw Western coaches and athletes begin to incorporate the use of performance enhancing drugs as part of event preparations (Voy, 1991; Yesalis & Bahrke, 2002).

The West took a very different approach. Despite recognition that a failure to engage meaningfully with doping was impugning rather than supporting Western athletes, rhetoric typically criticised athletes consuming anabolic steroids as deviants determined to cheat no matter what (Hunt et al., 2014). It is unclear at what point doping by athletes became a taboo to be concealed from consumers in the West, but it may have had some basis in the mythologies emerging from the Cold War used to promote ideological supremacy (e.g. 'clean amateurs' from the West defeating 'doped professionals' from the East). That is, the West consolidated behind the idea that doping was against that which made sport intrinsically valuable and therefore had no place in amateur sport.

The war begins in earnest

It is within this ideological context that the management of drugs in sport transitioned from an ideological to a very real war. Amateur sport introduced detection-based deterrence drug testing regimes at the 1968 Winter and Summer Olympic Games (Mazanov & McDermott, 2009). This 'detect and punish' approach became the foundation for drug control in amateur sport, including athletes forfeiting medals, prize money and eligibility to compete if they tested positive to a prohibited substance. The first medal forfeited for doping was a bronze medal awarded to Swedish modern pentathlete Hans-Gunnar Liljenwall for having 'two beers' to calm his nerves before the shooting discipline at the 1968 Summer Games (Rosen, 2008). The 'war on drugs in sport' had begun in earnest.

Poor management of drugs in sport

Managerial responses to the 'war on drugs in sport' led to some bizarre practices. The prevailing approach from managers was to protect institutional interests (e.g. medal winning potential) by concealing drug use from sports authorities, who appeared to be quite happy to be deceived (Dimeo, 2007; Houlihan 2002). For example, sanctions arising from drug test positives were cynically seen as a punishment for being sloppy (e.g. failing to cycle steroids properly before an event) rather than a transgression of the formal rules or intrinsic spiritual value of sport (Voy, 1991).

The collective denial of drug consumption as part of sporting practice and unwillingness to develop meaningful drug control (Hunt, Dimeo, & Jedlicka, 2012) saw Western sport lose managerial control. This was demonstrated by the evolution of informal doping networks in Western countries (Hunt et al., 2014; Yesalis & Bahrke, 2002). In the absence of a coherent response from sporting institutions, managers of sports programmes and their athletes were left to navigate a perilous world of clandestine drug use, misuse and abuse. Some athletes were fortunate enough to find sympathetic medical practitioners, but most had to rely on a 'doping grapevine' for information about sports-related drug use. The informal knowledge base was developed by trial and error, with errors often leading to profound and sometimes tragic health consequences. Eventually, informal networks developed a critical mass of knowledge that was disseminated through documents such as the *Underground Steroid Handbook* (Duchaine, 1981). This tradition continued through the early twenty-first century with online communities building the informal knowledge base by reporting personal experiments with new substances (Andreasson & Johansson, 2015; Smith & Stewart, 2012). Indeed, some commentators have observed that the level of knowledge about anabolic steroids in such communities extends well beyond the published scientific literature (Brennan, Kanayama, & Pope, 2013).

Prohibition and weak drug control saw the black market for drugs in sport flourish in the West, with adolescents among the most aggressive users (Hunt et al. 2014). The potential for this black market saw organised crime move into the supply and distribution of drugs for sport (Kayser & Smith, 2008). By the early twenty-first century organised crime was alleged to be a dominant supplier of drugs to athletes in Australia (Australian Crime Commission, 2013), with estimates from Italy showing the black market for performance enhancing drugs in that country alone was worth many billions of euro (Paoli & Donati, 2014).

The initiative is lost

The post-war years defined the ideological, managerial and administrative bases of drug control in sport for the remainder of the twentieth century. Like alcohol, the ideological battle that started in the 1920s took decades to win and become the dominant form of drug control for sport. The prohibitionist approach to drug control for sport found support with the 'war on drugs' thinking of the 1950s and 1960s.

What was missing was a coherent response from managers. Instead of building on the drug control systems put in place by professional sport and Soviet bloc sports managers, considerable effort was invested in preserving the fiction that elite Western sport was practised by 'clean amateurs'.

The end of the Cold War brought with it the end of formal state-sponsored doping. The sharp distinction between amateur and professional sport left only one option; the informal networks designed to conceal drug use in sport of the West became the dominant approach to managing drugs in sport. Sport had lost the initiative for the remainder of the twentieth century, and would only regain the initiative through a massive investment in the early twenty-first century.

Tobacco sponsorship: sport continues to lose the initiative

The 1950s saw the emergence of public health data that demonstrated a link between smoking and increased cancer risk. The following decade saw Western governments begin a co-ordinated effort to reduce smoking rates using a combination of medical and marketing restrictions. The medical efforts focused on overcoming the addictive properties of tobacco use, and the marketing restrictions were designed to prevent adolescents and young adults from starting. The 1960s prohibition of cigarette brand advertising in the United Kingdom sparked similar legislation around the world over the ensuing decades.

Tobacco companies quickly recognised ways to circumvent these laws through sports sponsorship of televised events (Hanstad & Waddington, 2009). The most prominent of these were naming rights sponsorships of competitions or leagues, which gave access to third party advertising (e.g. news broadcasts). In particular, tobacco companies cornered sponsorship markets in motor racing, horse racing, snooker and various forms of football (soccer and rugby league).

As the anti-cigarette movement gathered momentum through the later decades of the twentieth century, public health campaigns stigmatised cigarette smoking in the Industrialised West. This stigmatisation was achieved by, among other things, pointing out the harms cigarette smokers imposed on non-smokers through 'passive smoking', the impact of smoking while pregnant (e.g. low birth weights), or characterising smokers as absorbing a disproportionate level of health resources. Tobacco sponsorship of sport to market cigarette smoking to children (Meier, 1991) became a deepening violation of both rules-based (marketing to children; e.g. Macklin & Carlson, 1999) and values-based expectations (the nexus between sport and health; see Chapter 10). For example, athletes caught smoking cigarettes have been demonised for promoting smoking among children (e.g. Elliott, 2010). Ongoing cigarette brand sponsorship of sport became increasingly out of step with prevailing views on cigarettes among consumers.

Despite increasing public opposition and government regulation of tobacco advertising, sports managers refused to 'kick the big tobacco sponsorship habit' (cf. Blum, 2005). Instead of seeking new sponsors that attracted far lower levels of regulation, ongoing inaction on tobacco sponsorship saw sports managers grow increasingly anxious about the financial future of their sports. Of course, history demonstrates that the sports in question survived the loss of tobacco sponsorship. By the early twenty-first century, tobacco sponsorship of sport had all but disappeared as First World governments imposed ever increasing restrictions around tobacco marketing and consumption (Crompton, 2014). Tobacco still finds significant sponsorship markets in the Developing World (e.g. Zimbabwe and East Timor) despite World Health Organisation treaty obligations to ban tobacco advertising.

The story of tobacco advertising regulation is an important element to drug control for sport. Part of the mythology of sport that made it intrinsically valuable was its social role as a moralising force and in producing natural, healthy citizens (muscular Christianity) (cf. Hanstad & Waddington, 2009). Tobacco clearly contravened those roles. Inaction by sports managers saw sport lose the initiative in controlling its relationship with tobacco sponsors. Where sport refused to adapt to the changing norms around tobacco, governments seized the initiative through regulation of tobacco advertising. This signalled a willingness among governments to impose drug control in the public interest where sports were reluctant to do so voluntarily. This becomes an essential part of sport drug control's story where governments take a controlling role in the formalisation of the anti-doping policy in the early twenty-first century.

Lost initiative: drug scandals and reactionary crisis management

As Olympic sport was losing the initiative with control of drugs, it was also going through fundamental changes, with the demise of amateurism, the rise of the Olympics as a global mega-event and increasing revenues. The new status of Olympic sport as very big business compelled the transition from amateur to professional management of sport. Several governance scandals demonstrated that adjusting to this new role took the International Olympic Committee some time (e.g. the Salt Lake bid scandal; Crowther, 2002; Wenn, Barney, & Martyn, 2011). This included the increasing interest in the management of sport by governments looking to respond to the growing hegemony of the International Olympic Committee. The failure to effectively manage relations with governments saw sport once again lose the initiative in its attempt to control management of drugs in sport.

The formalisation of drug control in sport emerged as a function of reactionary crisis management (Houlihan, 1999; Hunt *et al.*, 2012; Ritchie & Jackson, 2014). While the concealment strategy could cope with the occasional scandal, it was the concatenation of scandals and an increasing interest in the public health implications of sport that saw governments force sport to formalise drug control through the 1990s. A key problem was that concealment became more difficult as drug testing became more reliable. This led to a number of minor doping scandals across Australia, Canada, Germany and the United Kingdom (see Ritchie, 2013). These minor scandals 'primed the pump', such that the Ben Johnson sanction became the catalyst for sport working to regain managerial control over drug use. The Dubin Inquiry of Canada and the Black Inquiry in Australia became watersheds as both governments and the public became aware of the extent of the deception around drug use in sport. It took yet another series of scandals (e.g. the 1998 Tour de France and the 1998 World Swimming Championships) to demonstrate that control over the role of drugs in sport had been lost (Wagner & Pedersen, 2014). As a result, both sporting institutions and governments were finally motivated to work towards regaining the initiative by resourcing the World Anti-Doping Agency (WADA).

Regaining the initiative: the rise of anti-doping

WADA was founded after a particularly bruising encounter between the IOC and a series of governments at a 1999 conference in Lausanne. Put simply, the IOC underestimated the interest of the world's governments in the management of drugs in sport. Instead of being permitted to extend its hegemony to managing drugs in sport, the IOC was forced to share control with international governments (Hanstad, Smith, & Waddington, 2008). This is reflected in the funding arrangements (where half of WADA's funding comes from the IOC and the other half from governments across the world) and the composition of WADA Boards (again, half from the IOC and half from governments) (see Chapter 7).

Punitive prohibition was chosen as the overarching policy paradigm. This was perhaps an odd choice given the standing evidence for the failure of punitive prohibition both outside sport (e.g. alcohol prohibition) and inside sport (e.g. proliferation of doping). However, the politics emerging from the historical legacies of sport (e.g. moralising of drugs in sport) and broader drug control (e.g. the war on drugs) make the choice seem inevitable. It can only be presumed that governments assumed the failure of punitive prohibition up to the foundation of WADA lay in poor management (the mutual deception game) rather than the underlying ideology of the anti-doping policy. As a result, the decision was taken to keep the ideological basis of a punitive prohibitionist policy and focus efforts on improving the management of drugs in sport. As a result, drug control in sport was governed by a policy that had its ideological roots in the 1920s, was given its administrative foundations in the 1960s and was updated by early twenty-first century management practices.

Following the establishment of WADA and the first World Anti-Doping Code (WADC) in 2003 (updated in 2004, 2009 and 2015), sport managed to regain some of the initiative in regards to drug control. The WADC achieved this by establishing WADA as the sole arbiter with exclusive control over drug control in sport (see Chapter 7). The fact that the WADC confines potential opposition (e.g. Article 21.2.3 obliges athlete support personnel to promote attitudes consistent with anti-doping) reinforces the argument of a prevailing belief that the ideology underpinning punitive prohibition is sound (Jedlicka, 2014). WADA was granted a monopoly over drug control for sport using international conventions, treaties, processes and procedures. For example, the International Convention against Doping in Sport requires signatories to use their coercive powers in pursuit of punitive prohibition. This enables governments to legislate around doping, and set national and local policies relative to a standardised approach to managing drugs in sport (policy harmonisation). The IOC backed up the legislation by introducing requirements that entry of sports or athletes to Olympic events was contingent on WADC compliance. Equally, Olympic events could only be hosted by countries deemed to be compliant. The fact that so many powerful policy instruments were deployed gives an indication of just how profoundly sport had lost the initiative with drug control.

Regaining the initiative meant creating a sports drug control hegemony with WADA as the final authority (Jedlicka, 2014). The power of this hegemony became apparent following the collapse of the Fédération Internationale de Football Association resistance to various aspects of the WADC (Wagner, 2011). Major League Baseball experienced sustained political and media pressure in the wake of the Mitchell Report, resulting in eventual compromise towards drug control in line with the WADC. The hegemony has also extended to changing the management of drugs in non-Olympic professional sports. For example, the Australian Government threatened to withdraw financial support from the Australian Football League if it failed to achieve WADC compliance (Stewart et al., 2011).

Post anti-doping

Anti-doping significantly raised the profile of sports drug control, creating the conditions to regain the initiative. The ongoing debate around which drugs should appear on the Prohibited List demonstrates the range of drugs relevant to sport. Such debate reveals the extent to which drugs are an integral part of sport and why they need to be explicitly managed. Alongside the debate, the sensational sanctions of high-profile athletes (e.g. Lance Armstrong) and detection of drug users at consecutive Summer, Winter and Youth Olympics has led to an increased awareness of issues around drugs in sport in the general public (Engelberg, Moston, & Skinner, 2012; Solberg, Hanstad, & Thøring, 2010; Stamm, Lamprecht, Kamber, Marti, & Mahler, 2008). This awareness then translates into a generally understood sentiment that the role of drugs in sport needs to be managed. As a result, the WADC has had a significant influence on regaining the initiative over managing drugs in sport.

However, any suggestion that anti-doping has won the initiative with regards to management of drugs in sport is too ambitious. Like all policy paradigms, implementation has revealed a number of wicked problems arising from the WADC. A key problem is that while the frameworks designed to give effect to drug control at the institutional level have worked well, there is little evidence that they have improved drug control among sports practitioners (see Chapter 7). For example, there is evidence of significant variation in both the interpretation and implementation of the WADC across jurisdictions (Overbye & Wagner, 2014; Hanstad, Skille, & Loland, 2010). This resonates with the start of the war on drugs in sport, where punishment was meted out to those foolish enough to be caught rather than arresting drug-related harms. While this presents a problem for the WADC, the fact that these issues are explicit as part of the drug control debate creates the conditions for sport to regain the initiative.

Another wicked problem is that the WADC was designed to manage the role of performance enhancing drugs rather than as a system to manage drugs more generally. The regulation of illicit substances with performance enhancing potential (e.g. cocaine and amphetamines) appears to be consistent with the aims of the WADC. Problems arise when the WADC attempts to regulate illicit drugs with no performance enhancing potential (Welch, 2001). For example, the inclusion of marijuana as a prohibited substance with no performance enhancing implications has proven controversial (Waddington, Christiansen, Gleaves, Hoberman, & Møller, 2013). Equally, sports that adopt the WADC to manage doping may use a different approach for illicit drugs. For example, the Australian Football League seeks to treat athletes for drug misuse or abuse in the first instance, with sanctions applied if treatment is unsuccessful (Harcourt, Unglik, &

Cook, 2012). It is unclear whether the WADC or the illicit drugs policy should apply.

The emergence of wicked problems with anti-doping has led to development of alternative views on drug control for sport (see Chapters 4 and 12). The late twentieth and early twenty-first centuries saw rising interest in harm-minimisation approaches to manage the role of illicit drugs. Harm-minimisation argues that the main harms arising from drug misuse and abuse can be averted by treating the underlying problem of physical or psychological dependence. For example, harm-minimisation posits that sending a person with drug dependence to drug rehabilitation is likely to lead to better outcomes for the person and society, at least when measured against the harms to the person and society from sending them to prison. Applying such arguments to sport suggests that a sports drug control system should focus on ensuring athletes use drugs safely rather than exposing them to the harms of clandestine drug consumption seen in the West during the Cold War. While the debate has stagnated into polarised two-party oppositional defiance (see Chapter 1), the fact that the debate is occurring is a core indicator that anti-doping has led sport to regain at least some of the initiative when it comes to managing drugs in sport.

Potentially losing the initiative in the future

Two examples of managers failing to learn the lessons of history threaten sport's investment in anti-doping to regain control over drugs in sport. The first emerges from the apparent parallels in the relationship sport has had with the tobacco and alcohol industries. There are increasing concerns about direct (e.g. public health) and indirect (e.g. family breakdown) harms caused by alcohol, and how alcohol advertising is related to these harms. The evidence that alcohol advertising significantly influences adolescent alcohol consumption (Anderson, De Bruijn, Angus, Gordon, & Hastings, 2009) points to alcohol companies circumventing legislation restricting television advertising (especially to minors) in the interests of public health by becoming naming rights sponsors of sports events (see Chapter 10). Sports managers are becoming increasingly anxious about their capacity to attract similarly lucrative sponsors if they are prevented from accessing money from alcohol companies. History shows this anxiety is misplaced and that government will regulate if sport fails to voluntarily act in the public interest. That is, managers risk losing the initiative with alcohol control by focusing on short-term sponsorship outcomes rather than finding ways to work with the alcohol industry in the long term.

The second loss of initiative relates to the supplements market. Governments appear reluctant to regulate the supplements industry (discussed further in Chapter 8). On this basis, sports managers appear only too happy to link their brands with the health and performance claims attached to supplements. This is despite evidence that the misuse or abuse of supplements can be just as harmful as other regulated drugs, contamination of supplements with prescription drugs and claims that supplements are 'legal doping' (despite little evidence that supplements achieve the claims made in such advertising). Supplements represent an opportunity for sports to gain the initiative with drug control. This can be achieved by forcing supplements manufacturers to back their claims with independent evidence before linking with the brand or limiting the conditions under which an athlete can be sponsored by a supplements company.

Conclusion

The management of drugs in sport has had to reconcile romanticised notions of sporting virtues with the ugly reality of drug abuse. Sport lost the initiative to effectively manage the role of drugs with the clumsy attempt to conceal the role of drugs in sports production. Having lost the initiative, it has taken a significant level of investment by both governments and sports to regain at least some control. The investment to regain control has provided a platform from which to meaningfully debate drug controlled integrity management for sport. It remains to be seen whether a twentieth-century drug control policy responds effectively to the needs of twenty-first century sport.

Addendum

As drafting of the book drew to a close, a number of drug-related scandals for sport came to light. While the most sensational was Maria Sharapova's use of meldonium, the claims about systematic doping in Russia and China which raised concerns about the integrity of anti-doping were the most worrying. As the Independent Commission investigating doping in Russian athletics observed, it would be naive to think the problems were confined to either that country or that sport (Pound, McLaren, & Younger, 2015). In terms of the historical analysis of drug control for sport, this could be interpreted as a signal that sport may be losing the hard-won initiative.

References

Anderson, P., De Bruijn, A., Angus, K., Gordon, R., & Hastings, G. (2009). Impact of alcohol advertising and media exposure on adolescent alcohol use: a systematic review of longitudinal studies. *Alcohol and Alcoholism*, 44(3), 229–243.

Anderson, S., & Berridge, V. (2000). Opium in 20th-century Britain: pharmacists, regulation and the people. *Addiction*, 95(1), 23–36.

Andreasson, J., & Johansson, T. (2015). Online doping. The new self-help culture of ethnopharmacology. *Sport in Society*, DOI: 10.1080/17430437.2015.1096246

Australian Crime Commission (2013). Organised Crime and Drugs in Sport. Available at: www.crimecommission.gov.au/publications/intelligence-products/unclassified-strategic-assessments/organised-crime-and-drugs (accessed 12 February 2016).

Beamish, R., & Ritchie, I. (2004). From chivalrous 'brothers-in-arms' to the eligible athlete: changed principles and the IOC's banned substance list. *International Review for the Sociology of Sport*, 39(4), 355–371.

Bennett, D. (2013). Harm reduction and NFL drug policy. *Journal of Sport and Social Issues*, 37(2), 160–175.

Bergen-Cico, D. K. (2012). *War and Drugs: The Role of Military Conflict in the Development of Substance Abuse*. Abingdon: Routledge.

Bewley-Taylor, D. R. (2005). Emerging policy contradictions between the United Nations drug control system and the core values of the United Nations. *International Journal of Drug Policy*, 16(6), 423–431.

Blum, A. (2005). Tobacco in sport: An endless addiction? *Tobacco Control*, 14(1–2).

Brandt, A. M. (2007). *The Cigarette Century: The Rise, Fall, and Deadly Persistence of the Product that Defined America*. New York: Basic Books.

Breen, T. H. (2009). *Tobacco Culture: The Mentality of the Great Tidewater Planters on the Eve of Revolution*. Princeton, NJ: Princeton University Press.

Brennan, B. P., Kanayama, G., & Pope, H. G. (2013). Performance-Enhancing Drugs on the Web: A Growing Public-Health Issue. *The American Journal on Addictions*, 22(2), 158–161.

Brewer, B. D. (2002). Commercialization in Professional Cycling 1950–2001: Institutional Transformations and the Rationalization of 'Doping'. *Sociology of Sport Journal*, 19(3), 276–301.

Buescher, J. (2012). In the habit: A history of Catholicism and tobacco. Available at: www.catholicworldreport.com/Item/1762/in_the_habit_a_history_of_catholicism_and_tobacco.aspx (accessed 12 February 2016).

Burns, E. (2009). *The Smoke of the Gods: A Social History of Tobacco*. Philadelphia: Temple University Press.

Chrzan, J. (2013). *Alcohol: Social Drinking in Cultural Context*. Abingdon: Routledge.

Coomber, R. (2014). How social fear of drugs in the non-sporting world creates a framework for doping policy in the sporting world. *International Journal of Sport Policy and Politics*, 6(2), 171–193.

Crompton, J. L. (2014). Potential negative outcomes from sponsorship for a sport property. *Managing Leisure*, 19(6), 420–441.

Crowther, N. B. (1996). Athlete and State: Qualifying for the Olympic Games in Ancient Greece. *Journal of Sport History*, 23(1), 34–43.

Crowther, N. (2002). The Salt Lake City Scandals and the Ancient Olympic Games. *International Journal of the History of Sport*, 19(4), 169–178.

Devine, T. M. (1976). The Colonial Trades and Industrial Investment in Scotland, c. 1700–1815. *The Economic History Review*, 29(1), 1–13.

Dimeo, P. (2007). *A History of Drug Use in Sport 1876–1976: Beyond Good and Evil*. Abingdon: Routledge.

Duchaine, D. (1981). *The Original Underground Steroid Handbook*. Santa Monica, CA: OEM.

Elliott, J. (2010). Athletes attacked for smoking habits. Available at: www.bbc.co.uk/news/health-11323847 (accessed 27 January 2016).

Engelberg, T., Moston, S., & Skinner, J. (2012). Public perception of sport anti-doping policy in Australia. *Drugs: Education, Prevention and Policy, 19*(1), 84–87.

Gleaves, J. (2011). Doped professionals and clean amateurs: Amateurism's influence on the modern philosophy of anti-doping. *Journal of Sport History, 38*(2), 237–254.

Gleaves, J., & Llewellyn, M. (2014). Sport, drugs and amateurism: Tracing the real cultural origins of anti-doping rules in international sport. *The International Journal of the History of Sport, 31*(8), 839–853.

Goodman, J. (2005). *Tobacco in History: The Cultures of Dependence.* London: Routledge.

Hall, D. E. (Ed.). (1994). *Muscular Christianity: Embodying the Victorian Age.* Cambridge, UK: Cambridge University Press.

Hall, W. (2010). What are the policy lessons of National Alcohol Prohibition in the United States, 1920–1933? *Addiction, 105*(7), 1164–1173.

Hamm, R. F. (1995). *Shaping the Eighteenth Amendment: Temperance Reform, Legal Culture, and the Polity, 1880–1920.* Chapel Hill, NC: University of North Carolina Press.

Hanes, W. T., & Sanello, F. (2004). *Opium Wars: The Addiction of One Empire and the Corruption of Another.* Naperville, IL: Sourcebooks.

Hanstad, D. V., & Waddington, I. (2009). Sport, health and drugs: A critical re-examination of some key issues and problems. *Perspectives in Public Health, 129*(4), 174–182.

Hanstad, D. V., Smith, A., & Waddington, I. (2008). The establishment of the World Anti-Doping Agency: A study of the management of organizational change and unplanned outcomes. *International Review for the Sociology of Sport, 43*(3), 227–249.

Hanstad, D. V., Skille, E. Å., & Loland, S. (2010). Harmonization of anti-doping work: Myth or reality? *Sport in Society, 13*(3), 418–430.

Harcourt, P. R., Unglik, H., & Cook, J. L. (2012). A strategy to reduce illicit drug use is effective in elite Australian football. *British Journal of Sports Medicine, 46*(13), 943–945.

Herzberg, D. (2009). *Happy Pills in America: From Milltown to Prozac.* Baltimore, MD: Johns Hopkins University Press.

Hoberman, J. M. (1992). *Mortal Engines: The Science of Performance and the Dehumanisation of Sport.* New York: Free Press.

Houlihan, B. (1999). Anti-doping policy in sport: The politics of international policy co-ordination. *Public Administration, 77*(2), 311–334.

Houlihan, B. (2002). *Dying to Win* (2nd Ed.). Strasbourg: Council of Europe Publishing.

Hunt, T. M. (2007). Countering the Soviet threat in the Olympic medals race: The Amateur Sports Act of 1978 and American athletics policy reform. *International Journal of the History of Sport, 24*(6), 796–818.

Hunt, T. M., Dimeo, P., & Jedlicka, S. R. (2012). The historical roots of today's problems: A critical appraisal of the international anti-doping movement. *Performance Enhancement and Health, 1*(2), 55–60.

Hunt, T. M., Dimeo, P., Hemme, F., & Mueller, A. (2014). The health risks of doping during the Cold War: A comparative analysis of the two sides of the Iron Curtain. *International Journal of the History of Sport, 31*(17), 2230–2244.

Jedlicka, S. (2014). The normative discourse of anti-doping policy. *International Journal of Sport Policy and Politics, 6*(3), 429–442.

Kayser, B., & Smith, A. C. T. (2008). Globalisation of anti-doping: The reverse side of the medal. *British Medical Journal, 337*(7661), 85–87.

Kyle, D. (2015). *Sport and Spectacle in the Ancient World* (2nd Ed.). Chichester, UK: John Wiley & Sons.

Lee, M. A. (2012). *Smoke Signals: A Social History of Marijuana – Medical, Recreational and Scientific.* New York: Scribner.

Lee, M. A., & Shlain, B. (1985). *Acid Dreams: The Complete Social History of LSD: The CIA, the Sixties, and Beyond.* New York: Grove Press.

Leonard, J. (2001). Doping in elite swimming: A case study of the modern era from 1970 forward. In W. Wilson, & E. Derse (Eds.), *Doping in Elite Sport: The Politics of Drugs in the Olympic Movement* (pp. 225–239). Champaign, IL: Human Kinetics.

Lesch, W. C., & Middendorf-Brand, M. (1997). Cigarettes and health: Historical controversies and constraints – Part I. *Health Marketing Quarterly, 14*(3), 69–90.

Levine, H. G., & Reinarman, C. (1991). From prohibition to regulation: Lessons from alcohol policy for drug policy. *The Milbank Quarterly, 69*(3), 461–494.

López, B. (2014). Creating fear: the 'doping deaths', risk communication and the anti-doping campaign. *International Journal of Sport Policy and Politics, 6*(2), 213–225.

Lum, K. L., Polansky, J. R., Jackler, R. K., & Glantz, S. A. (2008). Signed, sealed and delivered: 'Big tobacco' in Hollywood, 1927–1951. *Tobacco Control, 17*(5), 313–323.

MacAloon, J. (Ed.). (2013). *Muscular Christianity and the Colonial and Post-Colonial World.* Abingdon: Routledge.

Macklin, M. C., & Carlson, L. (Eds.). (1999). *Advertising to Children: Concepts and Controversies.* Thousand Oaks, CA: Sage Publications.

Masteralexis, L. P. (2006). Drug testing provisions: An examination of disparities in rules and collective bargaining agreement provisions. *New England Law Review, 40*(3), 775–788.

Mazanov, J., & McDermott, V. (2009). The case for a social science of drugs in sport. *Sport in Society, 12*(3), 276–295.

Meier, K. S. (1991). Tobacco truths: the impact of role models on children's attitudes toward smoking. *Health Education and Behavior, 18*(2), 173–182.

Overbye, M., & Wagner, U. (2014). Experiences, attitudes and trust: An inquiry into elite athletes' perception of the whereabouts reporting system. *International Journal of Sport Policy and Politics, 6*(3), 407–428.

Paoli, L., & Donati, A. (2014). *The Sports Doping Market.* New York: Springer.

Porritt, A. (1965). Doping. *Olympic Review, 90*(May 1965), 47–49.

Pound, R., McLaren, R., & Younger, G. (2015). *Independent Commission Report #1.* Montreal: World Anti-Doping Agency.

Putney, C. (2001). *Muscular Christianity: Manhood and Sports in Protestant America, 1880–1920.* Cambridge, MA: Harvard University Press.

Rabushka, A. (2010). *Taxation in Colonial America.* Princeton, NJ: Princeton University Press.

Remijsen, S. (2015). The end of the ancient Olympics and other contests: why the agonistic circuit collapsed in late antiquity. *The Journal of Hellenic Studies*, *135*(January 2015), 147–164.

Ritchie, I. (2013). The construction of a policy: The World Anti-Doping Code's 'spirit of sport' clause. *Performance Enhancement and Health*, *2*(4), 194–200.

Ritchie, I. (2014). Pierre de Coubertin, doped 'amateurs' and the 'spirit of sport': the role of mythology in Olympic anti-doping policies. *International Journal of the History of Sport*, *31*(8), 820–838.

Ritchie, I., & Jackson, G. (2014). Politics and 'shock': reactionary anti-doping policy objectives in Canadian and international sport. *International Journal of Sport Policy and Politics*, *6*(2), 195–212.

Rosen, D. (2008). *Dope: A History of Performance Enhancement in Sports from the Nineteenth Century to Today*. Westport, CT: Praegar.

Smith, A., & Stewart, B. (2012). Body conceptions and virtual ethnopharmacology in an online bodybuilding community. *Performance Enhancement and Health*, *1*(1), 35–38.

Solberg, H. A., Hanstad, D. V., & Thøring, T. A. (2010). Doping in elite sport – do the fans care? Public opinion on the consequences of doping scandals. *International Journal of Sports Marketing and Sponsorship*, *11*(3), 2–16.

Stamm, H., Lamprecht, M., Kamber, M., Marti, B., & Mahler, N. (2008). The public perception of doping in sport in Switzerland, 1995–2004. *Journal of Sports Sciences*, *26*(3), 235–242.

Stewart, B., Adair, D., & Smith, A. (2011). Drivers of illicit drug use regulation in Australian sport. *Sport Management Review*, *14*(3), 237–245.

Ungerleider, S. (2001). *Faust's Gold: Inside the East German Doping Machine*. New York: Thomas Dunne.

Voy, R. (1991). *Drugs, Sport and Politics*. Champaign, IL: Human Kinetics.

Waddington, I., Christiansen, A. V., Gleaves, J., Hoberman, J., & Møller, V. (2013). Recreational drug use and sport: Time for a WADA rethink? *Performance Enhancement and Health*, *2*(2), 41–47.

Wagner, U. (2011). Towards the construction of the world anti-doping agency: Analyzing the approaches of FIFA and the IAAF to doping in sport. *European Sport Management Quarterly*, *11*(5), 445–470.

Wagner, U., & Pedersen, K. M. (2014). The IOC and the doping issue – An institutional discursive approach to organizational identity construction. *Sport Management Review*, *17*(2), 160–173.

Welch, R. (2001). A snort and a puff: Recreational drugs and discipline in professional sports. In J. O'Leary (Ed.), *Drugs and Doping in Sport: Sociolegal Perspectives* (pp. 75–90). London: Cavendish Publishing.

Wenn, S. R., Barney, R. K., & Martyn, S. G. (2011). *Tarnished Rings: The International Olympic Committee and the Salt Lake City Bid Scandal*. Syracuse, NY: Syracuse University Press.

Winter, J. C. (Ed.). (2000). *Tobacco use by Native North Americans: Sacred Smoke and Silent Killer*. Norman, OK: University of Oklahoma Press.

Yangwen, Z. (2005). *The Social Life of Opium in China*. Cambridge, UK: Cambridge University Press.

Yesalis, C. E., & Bahrke, M. S. (2002). History of doping in sport. *International Sports Studies*, *24*(1), 42–76.

Chapter 4

Policy context for managing drugs in sport

The history of drug control for sport shows that anti-doping became the dominant policy for managing drugs in sport (see Chapter 3). It is therefore essential to understand the principles underlying the dominant policy when considering drug control-led integrity management for sport. However, it would be a mistake to assume that anti-doping is the only policy available to drug control for sport. It is therefore equally essential for managers to understand the implications associated with policy alternatives. This becomes especially important should policy change, either through changes in societal views on drug control or sports managers using their influence to shape drug control policy for sport (Mazanov, 2013). The anti-doping policy is described and critiqued in detail, followed by a five-stage drug control model which is used to explore policy alternatives to anti-doping.

The anti-doping policy

The cornerstone of the anti-doping policy is the World Anti-Doping Code (the Code). It is the standard referred to by international conventions (e.g. the International Convention against Doping in Sport from the United Nations Educational, Scientific and Cultural Organization (UNESCO) and the Council of Europe's Anti-Doping Convention), international sports governing bodies (e.g. the IOC and FIFA) and sovereign governments. The Code is also the standard applied to contracts governing individual participation in sport, such as membership agreements with local sporting clubs. All references to the Code relate to the 2015 version.

From the outset, the Code establishes its purpose in terms of athlete health and sports integrity (specifically, fairness and equality) to preserve 'doping-free sport' (note that doping is defined in Article 2 of the Code; see below). The moral basis for protecting athlete health and sports integrity is defined through the Spirit of Sport statement (see Chapter 6). The Spirit statement presents 11 values that form the basis of Olympism and define that which is intrinsically valuable about sport (see Table 6.1). Doping is defined as contrary to the Spirit of Sport. It is with this justification that the Code elaborates how drug control for sport should occur.

Drug control for sport follows the legalistic prohibitionist approach (Waddington, 2000), consistent with the evolution of international efforts to control illicit drugs through the second half of the twentieth century (e.g. the United Nations). This approach sets out a system that describes how transgressions of specific rules are to be investigated and prosecuted, and if a transgression has occurred, the consequences of those transgressions. Under deterrence theory, these consequences needed to be severe enough to deter others from engaging in the same behaviour (Matthews & Agnew, 2008). The result is a system where athletes and their support personnel can be banned from sport for their complicity in 'doping'.

The anti-doping policy also seeks to implement the idea of 'policy harmonisation'. Harmonisation emerges when anti-doping is experienced the same way independently of geography or event. That is, policy harmonisation aims to avoid potential inconsistencies across countries and different types of sport, which is necessary to enable international sporting events such as the Olympic Games (Houlihan, 1999).

The Code defines 'doping' as an anti-doping rule violation (ADRV), with ten described under Article 2 of the Code (see Table 4.1). The first

Table 4.1 World anti-doping code article 2 anti-doping rule violations

Article	Description
2.1	Presence of a prohibited substance or its metabolites or markers in an athlete's sample
2.2	Use or attempted use by an athlete of a prohibited substance or a prohibited method
2.3	Evading, refusing or failing to submit to sample collection
2.4	Whereabouts failures
2.5	Tampering or attempted tampering with any part of doping control
2.6	Possession of a prohibited substance or a prohibited method
2.7	Trafficking or attempted trafficking in any prohibited substance or prohibited method
2.8	Administration or attempted administration to any athlete in-competition of any prohibited substance or prohibited method, or administration or attempted administration to any athlete out-of-competition of any prohibited substance or any prohibited method that is prohibited out-of-competition
2.9	Complicity
2.10	Prohibited association

two relate to athlete consumption of a prohibited drug. The remaining ADRVs become progressively removed from athlete drug consumption towards preserving the integrity of administrative systems (e.g. athlete availability for out-of-competition drug testing) and other behaviours deemed to influence athlete drug consumption (e.g. training with people who have been sanctioned). Note that it is possible for an athlete to be banned from sport for life despite never having contact with drugs. Equally, it is possible for an athlete support person (e.g. a sports trainer) to be banned from sport for life despite never having any contact with prohibited drugs.

Drugs are entered on to the Prohibited List when they meet at least two of three criteria outlined under Article 4.3. The first test relies upon evidence (including experience) that the drug enhances or has the potential to enhance sports performance. The second test is evidence (including experience) that the drug represents an actual or potential health risk to athletes. The third test is whether the drug is felt to violate the Spirit of Sport. Drugs can also appear on the Prohibited List if they are declared a potential 'masking agent', which identifies the drug as one which may interfere with the efficacy of tests designed to detect other drugs on the Prohibited List. Given prohibited drugs can also have legitimate therapeutic uses (e.g. anabolic steroids for muscle injuries), athletes and support personnel can be granted 'Therapeutic Use Exemptions' for illness or injury.

There are two types of investigation; analytic and non-analytic. Analytic investigations rely on a rigorous drug testing procedure. Early attempts at drug testing athletes for anti-doping led to a range of legal challenges that forced drug testing to mature into a robust process (e.g. Buti & Fridman, 1994; Fogel, 2014). Strict chain of custody procedures transfer samples to accredited laboratories that then perform objective probabilistic tests to determine the likelihood that a sample contains a prohibited drug. Non-analytic investigations rely on circumstantial evidence to build a case that an ADRV has occurred. For example, Lance Armstrong was banned from sport for life as a result of a combination of witness testimony and other evidence (USADA, 2012).

Both forms of investigation are prosecuted before a tribunal, formed by the sport or outsourced to an anti-doping organisation (e.g. WADA). The outcome of the tribunal can be appealed to the Court of Arbitration for Sport (CAS). The CAS is a tribunal that the parties have agreed will be the final avenue of appeal as part of the overarching agreement to be Code compliant. A range of factors can be taken into account in relation to sanctions, with four year (first offence) or life bans (second offence) from sport the default sanctions.

The Code sets out the roles and responsibilities for stakeholders in sport. The role and responsibilities for institutional stakeholders are outlined, such as the international and national Olympic committees. These include appropriate resourcing and educating athletes and support personnel about their obligations under the Code. It also sets out the roles and responsibilities for individuals, proscribing expectations of athletes and athlete support personnel such as using their influence to promote the Code.

The anti-doping policy uses the legalistic prohibitionist approach to regulate drug consumption and behaviours related to drug consumption through a system of detection, prosecution and sanction. In doing so, it sets out clear guidance for what counts as sport (only those that comply with the Code can be considered legitimate sports) and who can participate in those sports (Jedlicka, 2014). As the incumbent policy, it is unsurprising the anti-doping policy has attracted significant criticism.

Critiques of the anti-doping policy

Almost every aspect of the anti-doping policy has been critiqued in some form, leading both academics and WADA itself to declare the anti-doping policy a failure (see Engelberg, Moston, & Skinner, 2015, p. 269). Given the depth of critiques, an overview mirroring the description of the anti-doping policy is presented.

The anti-doping hegemony

Jedlicka (2014) argues that the Code has been written in such a way as to brook no challenge, and that those who would be part of sport are expected to engage in happy and silent obedience to the authority of WADA (p. 439). This approach is reflected in research programmes run by anti-doping organisations which require research to 'promote anti-doping', meaning research which potentially contradicts anti-doping is never funded (Møller & Dimeo, 2014). For example, studies establishing safety data for elite athletes using erythropoietin or anabolic steroids are prevented under the International Convention against Doping in Sport. This active prevention of policy alternatives contradicts the basis of policy development and robust democracy (Althaus, Bridgman, & Davis, 2013).

Health, fairness and equality

The Code has been criticised for failing to protect athlete health. For example, athletes have been denied therapeutic use exemptions for drugs that enable their participation in sport; a cyclist taking medically supervised supplemental testosterone for hypogonadism was denied an exemption (Henning & Dimeo, 2015). Fairness is often constructed as a function of the assumed distorting effects of performance enhancing drugs on competition, with prohibition aimed at protecting the 'level playing field'.

Unfortunately, other factors distort competition far more than drugs, with athletes from wealthy industrial nations winning the majority of medals in Olympic competition (Celik & Gius, 2014; Houlihan, 2002); thus, performance enhancing drugs potentially distort which wealthy industrial nation wins rather than resolving fundamental challenges to the level playing field. Equality is problematic in the sense that sanctions have differential effects on different athletes (Amos & Fridman, 2009; see Chapter 11). For example, bans may end the career of a female gymnast while being a potentially valuable hiatus for cyclists or football/soccer players (e.g. injury recovery and technical training).

Spirit of Sport

The Code provides no guidance on what the Spirit of Sport values actually mean. Some argue that this is a strength in the Code, allowing the ethical basis for sport to be universally understood as subtle variations of the 11 values (McNamee, 2012). Others argue that the failure to provide a more precise definition is sociologically naive and increases the risks of athlete exploitation, calling for the Spirit statement to be operationalised more fully to enable a richer realisation for the justification of anti-doping (Loland & Hoppeler, 2012; Mazanov & Huybers, 2016). The failure to provide guidance on what the values mean creates room for creative reinterpretation of the Spirit statement to suit a range of arguments. For example, some critics of anti-doping use the Spirit statement to demonstrate ethical contradictions in the Code (Savulescu, Foddy, & Clayton, 2004). More practically, the ethical ambiguity can become problematic when athletes ask managers or mentors why they should comply with the Code. This potential weakness in the Code raises uncertainty about the ethical justification for anti-doping to protect the integrity of sport from drug-related harms. Robust debate about whether the Spirit statement represents what is intrinsically valuable about sport is needed (see Chapter 6).

The failure of deterrence theory

The failure for the Code to have a meaningful deterrent effect has been argued to be a consequence of the perceived likelihood of detection being very low (Engelberg et al., 2015). Put simply, athletes maintain a belief that the chances of being caught are so low that seeing another athlete sanctioned has no impact on their behaviour.

Policy harmonisation

The early evidence suggests mixed results for policy harmonisation. There has been significant success in getting almost universal agreement to adopt and comply with the Code (Houlihan, 2014). However, this success has been undermined by significant variation in how the Code has been interpreted and supported in local contexts (Hanstad, Skille, & Loland, 2010). For example, while wealthy countries can afford to establish and resource anti-doping organisations, less wealthy countries (e.g. Jamaica and Kenya) may focus resources on nation building rather than drug control for sport (Kayser, Maruon, & Miah, 2007). The challenge for policy harmonisation is also apparent in wealthy countries, where European athletes observe significant differences in how anti-doping is implemented across national boundaries (Overbye and Wagner, 2014). That being said, at the time of writing the Code was still a relatively young policy with ongoing investment of resources looking to overcome the challenges of policy harmonisation.

Definition of doping

The Code's definition of doping goes well beyond sport and well beyond drug control. The direct effect can be observed by the vigorous debate about whether illicit drugs with no performance enhancing implications, marijuana is used as the exemplar, should be eligible to be prohibited under the Code (Waddington, Christiansen, Gleaves, Hoberman, & Møller, 2013). The debate focuses around whether the Code oversteps its boundaries by regulating drug use among athletes and support personnel outside of sport. For example, an American judoka was sanctioned for consuming a 'marijuana brownie' well before the London Games (IOC, 2012); the debate seeks to resolve whether such sanctions are legitimate given the aims of the anti-doping policy. The Code also appears to be creeping towards broader regulation of integrity in society across degrees of separation from sport, such that a person who has never agreed to comply can still be sanctioned. For example, under Article 2.10, a person serving a criminal conviction for trafficking prohibited veterinary steroids to farmers can be deemed to have committed an ADRV. The Code's expanding sphere of influence regulating integrity well beyond both sport and drugs has also been demonstrated in debate around regulating performance enhancing technologies outside sport (see Chapter 1). As a result, it would be a mistake to think the anti-doping policy's influence is limited to drug control in sport.

Prohibition tests

The three tests underpinning prohibition merit deeper investigation as the clearest expression of what the anti-doping policy seeks to achieve and the foundation to the ADRV. The inclusion of the 'experience' criterion suggests that a drug could be considered performance enhancing or injurious based on a socially constructed exaggeration of effects (Coomber, 2014; Crichter, 2013). This appears to have been the case for erythropoietin, with credible evidence discounted in favour of a moral panic around the drug (López, 2011).

When evidence is brought to bear, the way drugs are defined as having performance enhancing or health implications is also problematic. The evidence shows that some drugs appearing on the Prohibited List have highly variable performance enhancing effects, have little performance enhancing effect or actually impair performance. For example, assessment of Major League Baseball pitchers known to have used anabolic-androgenic steroids demonstrates little increase in fast ball velocity; instead, the use of such steroids appears to prolong the career of pitchers (Addona and Roth, 2010). Further, human growth hormone appeared to have a negative impact on fast ball velocity.

The health test appears to prioritise physiological integrity using Western medicalised interpretations of health. This creates three problems. The first is that Western medicine can fail to account for the importance of spiritual health in many cultures (Haque, 2010), such as when a prohibited drug is intrinsic to spiritual health (e.g. the Rastafari Movement). The second is that drugs with mental or social health implications may be absent from the Prohibited List; such as prescription drugs consumed as narcotic substitutes or drugs of dependence (e.g. depressants or stimulants). The third draws on Chapter 2, where athletes may be denied *use* of a drug that protects their health in sporting contexts due to health risks associated with *misuse* or *abuse*.

Finally, the Spirit test was included as a 'catch-all', relying on the ambiguity of the Spirit statement to allow any drug meeting either of the performance or health tests, rather than both, to be prohibited (Ritchie, 2013). The combined effect of these tests is that a drug can be prohibited in the absence of objective evidence, which appears to contradict notions of integrity in sports systems that the anti-doping policy seeks to preserve.

Investigation

Analytic investigations are hampered by two key problems. The first is known as the 'doping arms race' (Mazanov & McDermott, 2009), where drug test development lags behind drug innovation. Attempts have been made to overcome this by securing agreements with large pharmaceutical companies (Rabin, 2011), although smaller scale drug development, such as that seen in the Bay Area Laboratory Co-operative (BALCO) case, means the arms race continues. The second is the sensitivity and specificity of drug tests. Challenges to drug testing on biostatistical (Berry, 2008; Pitsch, 2009), measurement (Van der Veen, 2003) and efficacy (Hermann & Henneberg, 2014) grounds have led to observations by WADA officials that drugs tests are of limited value (Pound, Ayotte, Parkinson, Pengilly, & Ryan, 2013), and perhaps why the anti-doping policy appears to have had little deterrent impact.

The increasingly apparent difficulties with objective drug testing have seen increasing enthusiasm for non-analytic investigations. Prosecution relies on the 'comfortable satisfaction' test, which sits between 'beyond reasonable doubt' and 'balance of probabilities'. There is debate around whether comfortable satisfaction is the right test given the profound implications of being sanctioned (e.g. losing the ability to derive an income) (Kornbeck, 2015; Morgan, 2006). Unfortunately, like drug tests, it appears the risk of being sanctioned as a result of a non-analytic investigation also has little deterrent impact (Huybers & Mazanov, 2012).

Roles and responsibilities

As noted in the discussion on policy harmonisation, the Code has been remarkably successful in terms of getting institutions to sign up. Unfortunately, there is no evidence the institutions are meeting their obligations, especially at the level of practice. For example, there is little evidence that sports organisations are resourcing anti-doping education leading to a profound level of ignorance about the Code among support personnel (see Chapter 9). Thus, it appears institutions are failing to meet their responsibilities to provide the supporting architecture to translate the Code from policy to practice, preventing athletes and support personnel from being able to meet their obligations. This point is discussed in more detail in Chapter 7.

Status of the anti-doping policy

The Code is an understandable response to the drug management crisis sport found itself in towards the end of the twentieth century, and a potentially necessary step to regain the initiative around sports drug control. It offers an elegant framework with which to advance the anti-doping ideology using the twin policy paradigms of legalistic prohibition and policy harmonisation. While the anti-doping ideology gestated for much of the twentieth century, it is still relatively young policy in terms of implementation. The transition from ideology to policy and the parallel critiques of that process demonstrate a great deal was learned about drug control for sport in a relatively short time (around a decade).

As argued by Mazanov and Connor (2010), the anti-doping policy has its greatest value as the first policy experiment around drug control for sport. The lessons learned from combining the twin paradigms inform other approaches to manage the role of drugs in sport. Given this experience, it is perhaps time to start exploiting the initiative earned by the anti-doping hegemony (see Chapter 3) to regain control over the management of drugs in sport by exploring policy alternatives using a five step continuum.

Alternatives to the anti-doping policy

The policy alternatives to anti-doping are explored using a continuum representing degrees of control from prohibition to permissiveness. The continuum is operationalised drawing on five general categories. First, a total control policy would see consumption of anything defined as a drug (see Chapter 2) result in permanent exclusion from all forms of sport. One step removed from uncompromising prohibition is a mixed system where the use of prohibited drugs has punitive consequences while the use of other drugs is permitted. The anti-doping policy fits in this general category. The next step along from anti-doping is a mixed system that seeks to control the use of drugs without punishing their use, one version of which is health-based harm-minimisation. The fourth category regulates the consequences rather than the use of drugs, presented here as a handicap system. The final category represents the absence of drug control, described by some as laissez-faire or 'open slather' (Mazanov, 2014).

Each point on the continuum is summarised and critiqued in terms of drug control-led integrity management for sport. Much like anti-doping, experience with any policy along the continuum would reveal a range of wicked problems, where attempts to resolve one set of problems reveal another set of problems. This demonstrates the truism that no policy is going to be an ideal solution to mitigate integrity for sport concerns arising from drug control. Instead, like all questions for drug control, each point along the continuum simply emphasises different priorities (Weatherburn, 2008).

Prohibition

This approach to drug control for sport prohibits the consumption of any drug. Under this policy, the definition of what constitutes a drug is crucial. The key is to avoid the problems arising from prohibition of selected drugs which complicates the anti-doping policy. This approach says that athletes should be barred from any refined or pharmaceutically processed substance. The aim is to prevent athletes from using nutritional supplements as much as prescription or illicit drugs.

The definition of what constitutes a drug under this approach draws on three key arguments underpinning anti-doping. The first is athlete health. Athletes are required to abstain from all types of drug use, misuse or abuse. In theory, this mitigates any harms arising from both licit drugs (e.g. alcohol and tobacco) and illicit drugs (e.g. cocaine and marijuana).

The second is the notion of the level playing field. Anti-doping has failed to protect sport from drugs distorting the outcome of events, with athletes free to use drugs that enhance performance (e.g. caffeine). Prohibiting all forms of drug use removes drug-based distortions entirely. This then leads to the third key argument, naturalness. That is, the idea athletic performances should be a function of an athlete's genetic potential interacting with personal effort (Hemphill, 2009; Miah, 2004). Without access to drugs, athletic performances are theoretically driven by some combination of lifestyle factors (e.g. conditioning, training, nutrition and psychology) that are attributable to the genetic talents and efforts of the athlete rather than drugs. As a consequence, producers and consumers can trust in the integrity of sports events, at least in terms of drugs.

Managerially speaking, this would require only slight modification of the existing anti-doping administrative framework. Like anti-doping, the presence of a drug would be a strict liability offence. For example, a drug entering an athlete's system through contaminated meat (Møller & Dimeo, 2014; Thompson, 2015) would be irrelevant. Extending the idea of a therapeutic use exemption, athletes requiring a drug to recover from illness or injury would be disqualified from competition until the drugs and their effects have been demonstrated to have left their system. Athletes would be confined to using whole rather than processed foods. Under such a system, athletes may find it easier to live in communal facilities prior to competition.

The system is vulnerable to exploitation. The most obvious weakness is exploiting the definition of a drug. However, this is no worse than the definitional problems anti-doping confronts when permitting drugs that are performance enhancing (caffeine) and prohibiting drugs that are performance debilitating (marijuana) Drug prohibition might see the doping arms race change focus towards the development of genetically modified plants and animals for sporting purposes. This may lead to some public good outcomes, with genetically modified organisms that improve the human condition well outside sport (see Mazanov & Connor, 2010).

However, complete prohibition would never work given the ubiquitous nature of drugs in sport. In terms of athletic performance, prohibition would have significant implications for athletic performances and recovery. These would necessarily have an impact on the commercial value of sport to stakeholders external to production. Prohibition would also make commercial relationships with drug companies a clear violation of expectancies. Given sport's longstanding lucrative commercial relationships with alcohol and tobacco (see Chapter 10), and strengthening relationship with the supplements industry, it seems unlikely that sport would forgo such revenues to enact a total prohibition policy.

Mixed prohibition

The anti-doping policy is the base mixed punitive system, with drugs on the Prohibited List excluded from sport and, by implication, drugs absent from the Prohibited List condoned either implicitly (where a drug is yet to be assessed) or explicitly (where a prohibited drug is removed from the list). The alternative policy for managing drugs in sport using a mixed punitive system is to change the focus of punishment. Even as the first version of the Code was being drafted, there were concerns about the focus on punishing athletes while support personnel (e.g. coaches) driving the drug use were exempt from punishment (British Medical Association, 2002). The 2009 Code saw the introduction of punishments for athlete support personnel. However, given organisations appear willing to sacrifice athletes to anti-doping in pursuit of institutional success (Aubel & Ohl, 2014; Connor, 2009), it may be more effective to create institutional incentives to drive drug control for sport.

Camporesi and Knuckles (2014) propose that the anti-doping policy's punitive approach needs to learn lessons from efforts to regulate environmental sustainability. Their principal argument is that the burden for demonstrating integrity in sport should be shifted from regulators to the entities responsible for the damage. For example, chemical companies should be required to demonstrate their products are environmentally safe rather than awaiting a verdict from the regulator after the product has hit the market. Applying this principle to sport, they argue that drug control for sport should refocus on organisational penalties, and specifically sponsors. Doing so creates a set of incentives for sponsors and sports to comply with drug control. For sponsors, being fined for breaching drug control is an avoidable increase in the cost of sponsorship. For sports, being fined could very quickly make sponsorship unattractive. In theory, this should protect sport from violations in rules- and values-based expectations from producers and consumers.

Note that this alternative mixed punitive system still relies on the anti-doping policy, and is therefore vulnerable to all the critiques outlined for that policy in terms of protecting athlete health and integrity in sporting competition. Camporesi & Knuckles (2014) note wicked problems emerge from this approach. First, it requires more investment in expensive drug test development (Kayser et al., 2007; Lippi, Banfi, Franchini, & Guidi, 2008) and potentially intensifies the doping arms race. Second, interfering with the commercial arrangements within the sports sector has the potential to reduce the value of the sports market (see Chapter 10).

Mixed

Mixed models seek to achieve drug control by allowing athletes to consume drugs without necessarily punishing that consumption. This approach is best characterised by health-based harm-minimisation, which has been offered as the main alternative to the anti-doping policy (e.g. Anderson, 2013; Kayser & Broers, 2012; Kirkwood, 2009; Smith & Stewart, 2008; Stewart & Smith, 2014). Harm-minimisation is an approach drawn from evidence in the broader drug control literature (e.g. illicit drugs) that demonstrates that the harms associated with punitive systems can contribute to or exceed the harms associated with drug consumption in the first place (see Chapter 12). For example, harm-minimisation argues that the status of drugs as illicit drives a range of behaviours that create harms well beyond the consumer, including criminal behaviours such as burglary or assault. Refocusing efforts on treatment for misuse and abuse of drugs therefore reduces the burden of drugs on a society.

In sport, this approach acknowledges that drugs have a functional role to play in sport, both in terms of protecting athlete health (by preventing, or treating injury and illness) and in terms of performance enhancement. The aim of drug control in sport should therefore be ensuring drugs are *used* (as per Chapter 2) rather than *misused* or *abused*. Where misuse or abuse of a drug is detected, the athlete might be disqualified from competition until they are able to demonstrate they have overcome the issues that led to the misuse or abuse (e.g. fatigue, failure to cope or self-medicating mental illness). The length of disqualification depends on the drug concerned. For example, misuse of alcohol (a single binge session leading to alcohol poisoning) might see an athlete return to competition within a week, whereas an ongoing substance dependence disorder might mean the end of an athlete's career.

One way proposed to achieve this is to allow athletes to use drugs under medical supervision. Harm-minimisation advocates point out anti-doping forces athletes to consume drugs without adequate medical advice or ongoing medical monitoring (e.g. Kayser et al., 2007). They argue that medical supervision averts harms to athlete health through avoiding misuse or abuse of the full range of drugs, rather than just prescription drugs like anabolic steroids. Greater access to drugs also potentially improves athlete health in terms of preventing injury or illness (see Chapter 1). Fairness concerns are addressed by pointing out that differential access to drugs distorts the level playing field. Drugs are argued to create fairer competition, as each athlete determines which suite of drugs interacts best with their physiology (much like optimising nutrition).

Opponents of harm-minimisation raise concerns that medically supervised drug use would fail to mitigate drug misuse or abuse, or the temptation to engage in drug consumption outside the regulations imposed to make harm-minimisation work (Wiesing, 2011). Mazanov (2016) raises several ethical objections to harm-minimisation. The first is that while harm-minimisation addresses concerns for adult drug consumption in sport, it fails to address the integrity concerns that arise from drug consumption by children (e.g. coercion and drug exploitation). The second is that harm-minimisation may fail to lead to any less drug-related harm to athlete health than anti-doping. The third critique is that, like anti-doping, harm-minimisation appears to privilege Western medicalised versions of health. The final critique is the observation that the prioritisation of health may be inconsistent with how producers and consumers wish to construct sport. Mazanov also notes lingering concerns that medically supervised doping is a step towards renewing state-sponsored doping.

While the harm-minimisation approach is the most mature of the alternatives to anti-doping, it still needs further refinement before implementation (see Chapter 12). As a policy alternative, harm-minimisation potentially addresses the rules- and values-based expectations of producers and consumers, but only so long as those expectations put protecting athlete health at the centre of the sports trust relationship (Mazanov, Huybers, & Connor, 2011).

Mixed permissive

The fourth step transitions towards permissive approaches. Where the mixed model still focuses on third party control of drug consumption (medical supervision), the mixed permissive approach relaxes third party control and responds to the consequences of drug consumption. This policy approach seeks to manage drug control-led integrity by placing the onus on athletes to be responsible for their own drug consumption by creating a trade-off between health and performance. First, athletes must demonstrate the drugs they take have no injurious impact (e.g. relative to clinical trial data). Second, athletes who take drugs with performance implications are given a handicap before each event.

The mixed permissive policy combines the ideas of harm-minimisation's health focus with Camporesi and Knuckles (2014) refocusing on the entities responsible for the behaviour rather than the regulator. For example, athletes self-regulate through a variation of the Bird and Wagner's (1997) drug diary, where athletes present a record of the drugs they have taken and evidence of ongoing monitoring that demonstrates consumption has had no injurious impact on health. Entry to competition might be predicated on a drug test that demonstrates the only drugs in an athlete's system are those present in the diary, and to determine that the biological profile of the athlete is within known safety tolerances (Savulescu et al., 2004). Any substance detected by a drug test that is inconsistent with the diary (even if the substance is unknown) leads to the athlete being denied entry to the event. By the same token, a biological profile that suggests ongoing alcohol abuse might also see an athlete denied entry to competition. This is designed to encourage athletes to take drugs that protect health and avoid drugs that may compromise health. Doing so should meet producer and consumer expectations that the integrity of athlete welfare is being maintained.

Within competition, athletes are handicapped based on the known properties of the drugs in their system. One way to handle this is to declare the outcome of an event once drug corrected results have been established. For example, athletes with caffeine in their system might be given a 3 per cent time penalty. Another way is to handicap athletes at the start of the event. For example, an athlete who regularly consumes marijuana might be given additional points or start an event slightly earlier. Alternatively, teams might start each game or season with a negative score, or may only earn half the points either during or for winning an event.

In policy terms, this approach seems unrealistic given the potential delays for drug corrected results or the wicked problem of developing a workable handicap system. However, if this system attracted the same level of resourcing as the anti-doping policy it may well work. For example, the policy may see greater investment in identifying the performance implications for a range of drugs. It may also promote the search for drugs that enhance athlete health without having performance enhancing implications.

Permissive

The permissive approach represents the absence of drug control. Athletes would be free to use any drug or combination of drugs. While this policy is remarkable in the sense it is easy to conceptualise, the practicalities of the policy mean it is self-defeating. As argued by Mazanov (2014), a thought experiment of the permissive approach always leads back to regulation. For example, the permissive system should see an increase in the number of drug-related deaths among athletes. It remains to be seen at what point consumers abandon a sport due to an unacceptable death rate. Equally, consumers may abandon a sport if the drugs make athletes look abnormal. The participation base and therefore the consumer base may erode as parents discourage children from sports that require drugs in pursuit of athletic careers. At some point, sports managers would be forced to engage some kind of drug control policy to address consumer concerns. As a result, the permissive policy would be an exercise in rediscovering the reasons why drug control is necessary for sport.

Drug control policy alternatives for sport

The policy discussion does make one thing clear; the integrity of sport is contingent upon having some form of drug control. While it is easy to glibly state support for an absence of drug control or total prohibition, consumer responses mean neither approach is commercially sustainable. Like an athlete no longer having a choice about whether to use drugs, only which drug to use, the only choice for sport is which drug control policy to adopt. That policy needs to accord with the expectations of producers and consumers. The anti-doping policy has been shaped by and has shaped expectations over the better part of a century, which suggests that it is in the best position to meet those expectations. Whether the anti-doping policy is able to meet the expectations it has set is a different matter entirely.

While the anti-doping hegemony stifles debate around drug control policy alternatives for sport, the alternatives raise important questions for drug control-led integrity management. The most pressing question is whether the anti-doping policy, designed to address integrity of sport concerns arising from the effects of performance enhancing drugs, is the right policy framework to adequately deal with other drugs that also have implications for sport, such as alcohol, caffeine and marijuana. As part of this, it begs the question whether another policy might be no worse or potentially better than anti-doping with a similar level of investment. It is also naive of the anti-doping policy to think it is unable to learn from policy alternatives. For example, while the mixed permissive system is perhaps less realistic, the notion of a handicap system might create a more powerful set of incentives around drug consumption. The mixed approach suggests that athlete health should be the only priority in drug control for sport, a claim that sport needs to address at some point. If the anti-doping policy is going to continue to be the preferred policy to manage drug control-led integrity for sport, it is going to need to learn from the alternative approaches.

References

Addona, V., & Roth, J. (2010). Quantifying the effect of performance enhancing drug use on fastball velocity in Major League Baseball. *Journal of Quantitative Analysis in Sport*, 6(6).

Althaus, C., Bridgman, P., & Davis, G. (2013). *The Australian Policy Handbook* (5th Ed.). Sydney: Allen & Unwin.

Amos, A., & Fridman, S. (2009). Drugs in sport: the legal issues. *Sport in Society*, 12(3), 356–374.

Anderson, J. (2013). Doping, sport and the law: time for repeal of prohibition? *International Journal of Law in Context*, 9(2), 135–159.

Aubel, O., & Ohl, F. (2014). An alternative approach to the prevention of doping in cycling. *International Journal of Drug Policy*, 25(6), 1094–1102.

Berry, D. A. (2008). The science of doping. *Nature, 454*(7205), 692–693.

Bird, E. J., & Wagner, G. G. (1997). Sport as a common property resource. A solution to the dilemmas of doping. *Journal of Conflict Resolution, 41*(6), 749–766.

British Medical Association (2002). *Drugs in Sport: The Pressure to Perform.* London: BMJ Publishing Group.

Buti, A., & Fridman, S. (1994). The intersection of law and policy: Drug testing in sport. *Australian Journal of Public Administration, 53*(4), 489–507.

Camporesi, S., & Knuckles, J. A. (2014). Shifting the burden of proof in doping: Lessons from environmental sustainability applied to high performance sport. *Reflective Practice, 15*(1), 106–118.

Celik, O., & Gius, M. (2014). Estimating the determinants of Summer Olympic Game performance. *International Journal of Applied Economics, 11*(1), 39–47.

Connor, J. (2009). The athlete as widget: how exploitation explains elite sport. *Sport in Society, 12*(10), 1369–1377.

Coomber, R. (2014). How social fear of drugs in the non-sporting world creates a framework for doping policy in the sporting world. *International Journal of Sport Policy and Politics, 6*(2), 171–193.

Crichter, C. (2013). New perspectives on anti-doping policy: From moral panic to moral regulation. *International Journal of Sport Policy and Politics, 6*(2), 153–169.

Engelberg, T., Moston, S., & Skinner, J. (2015). The final frontier of anti-doping: A study of athletes who have committed doping violations. *Sport Management Review, 18*(2), 268–279.

Fogel, C. A. (2014). Manufacturing muscle: an overview of the history and legal aspects of doping in sport. *European Journal of Sport Studies, 2*(2), 7–15.

Hanstad, D. V., Skille, E. A., & Loland, S. (2010). Harmonization of anti-doping work: Myth or reality? *Sport in Society, 13*(3), 418–430.

Haque, A. (2010). Mental health concepts in Southeast Asia: Diagnostic considerations and treatment implications. *Psychology, Health and Medicine, 15*(2), 127–134.

Hemphill, D. (2009). Performance enhancement and drug control in sport: ethical considerations. *Sport in Society, 12*(3), 313–326.

Henning, A. D., & Dimeo, P. (2015). Questions of fairness and anti-doping in US cycling: The contrasting experiences of professionals and amateurs. *Drugs: Education, Prevention and Policy, 22*(5), 400–409.

Hermann, A., & Henneberg, M. (2014). Long term effects of doping in sporting records: 1886–2012. *Journal of Human Sport and Exercise, 9*(3), 727–743.

Houlihan, B. (1999). Policy harmonisation: The example of global anti-doping policy. *Journal of Sport Management, 13*(3), 197–215.

Houlihan, B. (2002). *Dying to Win* (2nd Ed.). Strasbourg: Council of Europe Publishing.

Houlihan, B. (2014). Achieving compliance in international anti-doping policy: An analysis of the 2009 World Anti-Doping Code. *Sport Management Review, 17*(3), 265–276.

Huybers, T., & Mazanov, J. (2012). What would Kim do: A choice study of projected athlete doping considerations. *Journal of Sport Management, 26*(4), 322–334.

IOC (2012). IOC Disciplinary Commission Decision Regarding Mr Nicholas Delpopolo. Available at www.olympic.org/Documents/Commissions_PDFfiles/Disciplinary_commission/London2012_Decision-Disciplinary-Commission-Delpopolo.pdf (accessed 13 February 2016).

Jedlicka, S. (2014). The normative discourse of anti-doping policy. *International Journal of Sport Policy and Politics*, 6(3), 429–442.

Kayser, B., & Broers, B. (2012). The Olympics and harm reduction? *Harm Reduction Journal*, 9(33).

Kayser, B., Mauron, A., & Miah, A. (2007). Current anti-doping policy: A critical appraisal. *BMC Medical Ethics*, 8(2).

Kirkwood, K. (2009). Considering harm reduction as the future of doping control policy in international sport. *Quest*, 61(2), 180–190.

Kornbeck, J. (2015). Private regulation and public trust: Why increased transparency could strengthen the fight against doping. *Deutsche Zeitschrift fur Sportmedizin*, 66(5), 121–127.

Lippi, G., Banfi, G., Franchini, M., & Guidi, G. C. (2008). New strategies for doping control. *Journal of Sports Sciences*, 26(5), 441–445.

Loland, S., & Hoppeler, H. (2012). Justifying anti-doping: The fair opportunity principle and the biology of performance enhancement. *European Journal of Sport Science*, 12(4), 347–353.

López, B. (2011). The invention of a 'drug of mass destruction': Deconstructing the EPO myth. *Sport in History*, 31(1), 84–109.

Matthews, S. K., & Agnew, R. (2008). Extending deterrence theory: Do delinquent peers condition the relationship between perceptions of getting caught and offending? *Journal of Research in Crime and Delinquency*, 45(2), 91–118.

Mazanov, J. (2013). The management of performance enhancing drugs in high performance sport. In P. Sotiriadou, & V. De Bossche (Eds.), *Managing High Performance Sport* (pp. 272–294). Abingdon: Routledge.

Mazanov, J. (2014). Drug control in sport: Who and how. In B. Stewart, & M. Burke (Eds.), *Drugs and Sport: Writings from the Edge* (pp. 33–71). Melbourne: Dry Ink Press.

Mazanov, J. (2016). Beyond anti-doping and harm minimisation: A stakeholder–corporate social responsibility approach to drug control for sport. *Journal of Medical Ethics*, 42(4), 220–223.

Mazanov, J., & McDermott, V. (2009). The case for a social science of drugs in sport. *Sport in Society*, 12(3), 276–295.

Mazanov, J., & Connor, J. (2010). Rethinking the management of drugs in sport. *International Journal of Sport Policy*, 2(1), 49–63.

Mazanov, J., & Huybers, T. (2016). Societal and athletes' perspectives on doping use in sport: The Spirit of Sport. In V. Barkoukis, L. Lazarus, & H. Tsorbatzoudis (Eds.), *The Psychology of Doping in Sport* (pp. 140–150). Oxon: Routledge.

Mazanov, J., Huybers, T., & Connor, J. (2011). Qualitative evidence of a primary intervention point for elite athlete doping. *Journal of Science and Medicine in Sport*, 14(2), 106–110.

McNamee, M. J. (2012). The spirit of sport and the medicalisation of anti-doping: Empirical and normative ethics. *Asian Bioethics Review*, 4(4), 374–392.

Miah, A. (2004). *Genetically modified athletes: Biomedical ethics, gene doping and sport*. London: Routledge.

Morgan, W. J. (2006). Fair is fair, or is it? A moral consideration of the doping wars in American sport. *Sport in Society, 9*(2), 177–198.

Møller, V., & Dimeo, P. (2014). Anti-doping – the end of sport. *International Journal of Sport Policy and Politics, 6*(2), 259–272.

Overbye, M., & Wagner, U. (2014). Experiences, attitudes and trust: An inquiry into elite athletes' perception of the whereabouts reporting system. *International Journal of Sport Policy and Politics, 6*(3), 407–428.

Pitsch, W. (2009). 'The science of doping' revisited: Fallacies of the current anti-doping regime. *European Journal of Sport Science, 9*(2), 87–95.

Pound, R. W., Ayotte, C., Parkinson, A., Pengilly, A., & Ryan, A. (2013). *Report to WADA Executive Committee on Lack of Effectiveness of Testing Programs*. Montreal: WADA.

Rabin, O. (2011). Involvement of the health industry in the fight against doping in sport. *Forensic Science International, 213*(1), 10–14.

Ritchie, I. (2013). The construction of a policy: The World Anti-Doping Code's 'spirit of sport' clause. *Performance Enhancement and Health, 2*(4), 194–200.

Savulescu, J., Foddy, B., & Clayton, M. (2004). Why we should allow performance enhancing drugs in sport. *British Journal of Sports Medicine, 38*(6), 666–670.

Smith, A. C. T., & Stewart, B. (2008). Drug policy in sport: Hidden assumptions and inherent contradictions. *Drug and Alcohol Review, 27*(2), 123–129.

Stewart. B., & Smith, A. (2014). *Rethinking Drugs in Sport*. Abingdon: Routledge.

Thompson, L. (2015). 'Not proven?' The curious case of the contaminated steak: a study of the Alberto Contador case and its implications for the 2015 World Anti-Doping Code. *Laws of the Game, 1*(1).

USADA (2012). *Report on Proceedings under the World Anti-Doping Code and the USADA Protocol; United States Anti-Doping Agency, Claimant v. Lance Armstrong, Respondent; Reasoned Decision of the United States Anti-Doping Agency on Disqualification and Ineligibility*. Colorado Springs: USADA.

Van der Veen, A. M. H. (2003). Measurement uncertainty and doping control in sport. *Accreditation and Quality Assurance, 8*(7), 334–339.

Waddington, I. (2000). *Sport, Drugs and Health*. London: E&FN Spon.

Waddington, I., Christiansen, A. V., Gleaves, J., Hoberman, J., & Møller, V. (2013). Recreational drug use and sport: Time for a WADA rethink? *Performance Enhancement and Health, 2*(2), 41–47.

Weatherburn, D. (2008). Dilemmas in harm minimisation. *Addiction, 104*(3), 335–339.

Weising, U. (2011). Should performance enhancing drugs in sport be legalised under medical supervision? *Sports Medicine, 41*(2), 167–176.

Part II

Management

Chapter 5

Drug control and the business of sport

The corporatisation of sport has seen changes in management practice from largely ad hoc 'kitchen cabinets' to the adaptation of accepted business practices from other market sectors (Donnelly, 2015). As a consequence, the management of integrity through drug control in sport should be understood in terms of sport's business interests. In doing so, like any market sector, sport's interest in managing drugs lies in efforts to avoid or arrest revenue destruction and promote revenue creation. Both profit-making and not-for-profit sporting institutions and corporations need to meet market expectations about production; failure to do so can have profound implications for revenue. The nature of market expectations can be understood in terms of corporate stakeholder responsibility (CSR). Where Chapter 1 identified that sport has a responsibility to manage the role of drugs, the current chapter begins to explore how that responsibility translates into practice and drives the deeper inquiry into the management of drugs as a method to protect the integrity of sport.

Structure of the sports industry

Foster, O'Reilly and Davila (2016) describe the structure of the sports industry using stakeholder groups with a legitimate interest in sport (noting that who or what can be considered a stakeholder is contested and therefore definitionally imprecise; Miles, 2012). The structure of the sports industry is adapted to account for some stakeholders drawn into the sports industry as a result of drugs, including the pharmaceutical and supplements industries, organised crime and gambling. Table 5.1 summarises the interests of internal and external stakeholder groups relative to drug control-led integrity management for sport. Two key implications can be drawn from this summary of stakeholders; reconciling competing stakeholder interests and revenue.

Table 5.1 Sports industry stakeholders and drug use/control

Stakeholder	Description	Example	Integrity management	Drug Management
Internal to sports production				
League	Professional sport entity with member-clubs, typically based in a country or region	National Hockey League, English Premier League	Creating structures to promote a consistent product in line with shareholder and market expectations	Adapting relationship with drugs to be consistent with private interests of their sport
Federation	Not-for-profit organisation responsible for sport and sport disciplines globally, or by country, state/province/ territory, or region	British Triathlon Association, Swimming Canada	Establish and police constitutive rules-based expectations for sports production	Define the relationship sport has with drugs in the interests of their sport
Association	Governing body (normally not-for-profit) that is not single-sport based	NCAA, Pop Warner Little Scholars	Establish and police rules-based expectations for sports participation	Defines the relationship member sports can have with drugs
Clubs/teams	Members of a league who field competitive team(s)	Denver Broncos, Cabramatta Soccer Club	Implementation of league structures and protection of club interests	Monitoring and management of relationship with drugs across departments
Athletes/players	Participants ranging from professional to amateur to recreational	Individuals	Preserving personal integrity relative to institutional structures with a mix of compliance and non-compliance	Monitoring and managements of personal drug consumption

Coaches	Manager who makes personnel and game strategy decisions	Individuals	Preserving personal and club integrity relative to institutional structures with a mix of compliance and non-compliance	Monitoring and managing relationship of athletes with drugs in relation to on-field performance
Agents	Representatives of players from professional agents to parents; can be a company or an individual	Creative Artists Agency, Boras Corporation	Acting in the best interests of individual athletes	Monitoring and management of compliance in relation to athlete integrity
Players' associations	Unions or collectives that represent large groups of players	UNI World Athletes, AFL Players Association	Acting in the best interests of members	Monitoring and management of compliance in relation to member and union integrity
Mega-events	A global competition or series of competitions where athletes or teams participate	Olympic Games, Rugby World Cup	Creating structures that promote an event consistent with rules- and values-based expectations	Define the relationship participants have with drugs in the interests of event
Events	A competition or series of competitions where athletes or teams participate.	Australian Open, New York City Marathon	Creating structures that promote an event consistent with rules- and values-based expectations	Define the relationship participants have with drugs in the interests of event
Facilities	Venues (stadiums, arenas, fields, pools, courts. etc.) where sport takes place	Melbourne Cricket Grounds, Yankee Stadium	Providing infrastructure consistent with rules- and values-based expectations	Infrastructure enables event drug management
Sports medicine	Physicians who work with athletes	British Association of Sport and Exercise Medicine	Preserving professional and personal integrity with a mix of compliance and non-compliance	Drug use consistent with professional, medical and sports ethics

continued

Table 5.1 Sports industry stakeholders and drug use/control

Stakeholder	Description	Example	Integrity management	Drug Management
Apparel and equipment providers	Apparel and equipment for sport participation	Nike, Adidas, Reebok, Trek, Speedo	Production and association consistent with rules- and values-based expectations within and across sectors	Influencing drug management to promote sales
Regulatory bodies (multi-sport organisations)	Associations and sport law organisations who regulate or defend by issue or cause	World Anti-Doping Agency, Code Red	Promotion of production relative to values-based expectations	Regulation, resourcing and policing of drugs relative to values
External to sports production				
Media organisations	Networks, radio, digital and other organisations who produce or diffuse sport content across media channels	Yahoo Sports, ESPN, Sky, BBC	Production of content that attracts viewing audiences	Reporting sports drug practices to other stakeholders
Corporate sponsors	Corporations who invest to associate with a sport property with the goal of achieving business outcomes	Coca-Cola, Budweiser, HSBC, Samsung	Association of product in places likely to maintain or improve revenue	Influencing drug management to promote sales
Governments	National, State, Provincial, Territorial, and Municipal governments	Russian Federation, Government of Maharashtra, Manchester City Council	Regulation and policing of sports production relative to public interest	Regulation, resourcing and policing of drugs in sport in public interest

Fans	People who follow a particular sport, league, club, event, or athlete with passion and interest	Individuals	Consuming sport and sports-related products consistent with personal rules- and values-expectations	Revealed preference with regards drugs in sport
Communities	Any population that is impacted by a sport property	Local residents of a mega-event host city	Acting in the best interests of the local community	Revealed preference on acceptable relationship between drugs and sport
Pharmaceutical industry	Corporations that manufacture, market and sell drugs	Pfizer, Novartis, Bayer, Roche	Creating drug markets in line with shareholder and market expectations	Quality control (active agent), education and distribution
Supplement industry	Corporations that manufacture, market and sell supplements	Swisse, GNC, Centrum	Creating supplements markets in line with shareholder and market expectations	Quality control (contamination), education and distribution
Organised crime	Organisations that exploit markets created by regulation	Cosa Nostra, Triads, Yakuza	Private interest profit maximisation	Overcoming supply barriers
Legal gambling	Corporations that offer gambling services in relation to sport	Ladbrokes, Bet365	Bets based on transparent compliance with rules-based expectations	Promoting sports with acceptable drug management

Competing interests

The breadth of stakeholders with an interest in drug control for sport raises a well-established management problem; it is difficult to discern how the multiple competing interests might be prioritised. As argued in Chapter 3, the interests of sport have come a distant second in the context of conflicts between corporate tobacco and governments. Table 5.1 also shows that there are many more institutional interests in managing drugs in sport than there are individual interests. For example, it can be very easy to miss the interests of athletes, fans or sports medicine. Indeed, the impression from the review of stakeholders is an implication that the institutional interests are prioritised at the expense of individual interests (see Chapter 7 for more on this point). Further, while it may be easy to dismiss the interests of organised crime as a stakeholder, the complexity of the doping supply chain (Fincouer, van de Ven, & Mulrooney, 2015) and volume of the black market for sports-related drugs (Paoli & Donati, 2014) compels the inclusion of organised crime as a stakeholder in the management of drugs in sport. This raises a very difficult question about how competing interests across the spectrum of stakeholders should be prioritised.

For the purposes of this discussion, the focus is on drug control for sport driven by a single overarching institution such as the World Anti-Doping Agency (WADA), or a World Sports Drug Agency (Mazanov, 2014; see Chapter 12). This is done for convenience, although the principles are scalable to different levels of business practice. For example, the principles that apply to a World Sports Drug Agency also apply to how interests in drug management might be prioritised in a club or athlete union.

The model used by WADA is an equal division of interests between a coalition of governments and the International Olympic Committee, representing sporting organisations; that is, anti-doping is administered as a public–private partnership with half the shares 'owned' by each sector. This means that only the views of government and the Olympic movement are prioritised, with all other views discounted (e.g. non-Olympic sport, athlete unions, corporate sponsors, pharmaceutical companies, player agents and fans). While some may argue the duumvirate is an acceptable prioritisation of interests (e.g. governments maintaining a check and balance representative of the plurality within member nation interests), the exclusion of all other stakeholders may be considered problematic by others (e.g. Mazanov, 2016). If anti-doping is to be considered the template for managing all types of drug use related to sport, this broadens the interest of the role of drugs in sport beyond governments and the Olympic movement considerably (e.g. non-Olympic sport and drug manufacturers). For example, drug manufacturers may take a significant interest in the processes underlying prohibition of a new sports-relevant drug given the implications for sales, and league officials the costs of implementing changes to drug control policy. Some consideration of alternative prioritisation is therefore appropriate.

One obvious answer is to declare all interests of equal value (cf. Mazanov, 2016). In contrast to the WADA duumvirate, the interests of athletes or fans would be given equal weighting to the interests of sporting institutions, broadcasters or sponsors. There are two options for implementing such an approach. The first is to form an adversarial 'drugs in sport parliament' with an equal number of representatives from each stakeholder voting on issues of drug control, although this would likely devolve into either a two-party system (where decisions represent the views of pre-determined majority coalitions) or rendered unworkable by minority parties (where decisions can be difficult to achieve). The second is to develop an administrative system which draws on independent panels to investigate issues of drug management in consultation with stakeholders, issuing determinations based on their investigations. Both approaches have the potential to become highly resource intensive (see below).

The alternative is that the interests of some stakeholders should be prioritised over others. This creates the problem of working through the basis upon which stakeholder interests should be prioritised. Stakeholder interests could be prioritised on an objective or subjective basis. Objective methods determine priorities by a mechanism that is theoretically resistant to vested interests. For example, the analytic hierarchy process indicates conducting research into the value and influence of stakeholders to determine weightings computationally (Hosseini & Brenner, 1992). Capturing the range of inter-stakeholder and intra-stakeholder values and influence in support of such a process would be computationally challenging given the dynamical complexity arising from the breadth of stakeholders. A different objective method is to marketise interests by creating shareholders rather than stakeholders to prioritise interests. Floating WADA as a public company with a share allocation would see interests prioritised based on how much each stakeholder was willing to pay to have their interests represented. Assuming the market leads to optimal outcomes (noting market failure is part of the optimisation process), then the prioritisation of stakeholder interests would be readily apparent. For example, this approach might see athletes develop portfolio-based coalitions to ensure their interests are prioritised and pharmaceutical manufacturers pass on the opportunity to have their interests represented.

Subjective methods prioritise interests on an ethical basis. For example, Chapters 1 and 6 present arguments that the interests of athletes should be given priority over other stakeholder interests. Alternative arguments could be mounted using other ethical principles, such as prioritising stakeholder interests on the basis of 'fairness' (Evans & Evans, 2014; Phillips, 1997). In contrast, some alternatives might be eliminated on ethical grounds. For example, arguing that those with the greatest financial stake in sport would potentially lead to the interests of those outside sport (e.g. organised crime, gambling and corporate sponsors) being given more weight than the interests of those inside sport (e.g. athletes, associations and events).

Like any industry, the size and structure of the sports industry creates complexity in the attempt to integrate stakeholder interests. The difficulty lies in the practical reality that, at some point, the interests of some stakeholders are likely to be compromised. The basis upon which interests are prioritised points very clearly to a need for deeper discussion around both the business ethics (see Chapter 6) and governance (see Chapter 7) of drug control-led management of integrity in sport.

Revenue

The revenue implications of drug control emerge as a second issue arising from the review of stakeholders. Both profit and not-for-profit sports organisations need revenue to either promote shareholder interests or to promote their cause, respectively. Drug control needs to be at least neutral and preferably positive with regards to overall revenue. In terms of revenue destruction, drug management needs to prevent loss of revenues associated with violations in consumer expectations about sports production. In terms of revenue creation, drug management needs to find new ways of incorporating drugs into sport in ways that promote the level of trust consumers have in producers. Of course, it is the combination of revenue destruction and creation that leads to the overall value of drug control to sport.

Revenue destruction

There is certainly an intuitive case to be made that drug management can have an impact on revenue destruction in sport, notably through different types of drug-related scandal (see Chapter 10). In terms of individual athletes, this can see the value of sports properties diminish significantly, as occurred when sponsors reacted to Michael Phelps being charged with driving under the influence of alcohol. In terms of organisations, scandals can see the loss of revenues for failing to manage drugs appropriately, such as when German public broadcasters pulled their coverage of the Tour de France amid concerns over how drugs issues were being handled (Solberg, Hanstad, & Thøring, 2010). It is also possible for drug suppliers to threaten sports revenue, especially when suppliers make unsubstantiated claims about the effects of sports drugs (a common problem for supplements) linked to sports brands (Heneghan et al., 2012; Outram & Stewart, 2015). Drugs can also lead to revenue destruction when they have adverse effects on athlete performance. This can occur through athletes misusing drugs that unintentionally interfere with their performance (e.g. sleeping aids or illicit drugs). It can also occur through so-called 'negative doping', where athletes are given drugs with the intention of interfering with on-field performance in the interest of gambling or strategising a season (e.g. losing matches to improve draft pick position for the following season) (Lippi, Sanchis-Gomar, & Banfi, 2012).

As a consequence, any administrative structure devised to support drug control must cost less than the potential revenue destruction. That is, drug control represents a form of insurance against losses that may be experienced from breaches in the producer–consumer trust relationship. For example, the global costs of administering anti-doping were estimated to have been at least US$500 million in 2013–2014 (Maennig, 2014). This represents a modest investment of global sports industry revenues (US$121 billion in 2010 and estimated to be US$145 billion in 2015; PWC, 2011). However, there has been no independent research examining the direct and/or indirect costs of doping to sport (e.g. gate receipts, broadcast audiences, sponsorship and merchandising) and no independent research that establishes the direct and/or indirect costs of anti-doping. As a result, it is unclear to what extent the investment in anti-doping has prevented revenue destruction. It would be incorrect to suggest that drug management has had no effect on insuring sport against revenue destruction, just as much as it is incorrect to suggest that drug management has had an effect; there is no evidence either way.

It is also relevant to consider the costs of drug management as a form of revenue destruction. For example, the three-year anti-doping case made against players at the Essendon Football Club in Australia had significant direct costs, such as the AU$2 million fine imposed on the club by the Australian Football League, the AU$200,000 fine for breaching workplace health and safety imposed by the Victorian Government and the legal costs for the players and club. However, the indirect costs lead to significant revenue implications for players (reduced or lost value), support staff (reputational harms), the club (weakened position within league and loss of finals revenues), the league (reduced broadcast and sponsorship value), broadcasters (price reductions for advertising during scheduled Essendon games), merchandisers (lower sales volumes) and the general public (diminished tax receipts from sports consumption). Indeed, the Australian Football League was highly concerned about the impact of the investigation on brand value and diminished 2013 grand final ticket sales (Gowthorp, Greenhow, & O'Brien, 2016).

There may be other forms of revenue destruction. For example, parents may divert their children into non-sport activities as a result of the Essendon prosecution breaching rules- or values-based expectations (e.g. perceived drug culture, confidence in administrators, or treatment of players). Given the correlation between sports participation and sports consumption (Bennett, Ferreira, Lee, & Polite, 2009; Summers & Johnson, 1999), this has the potential to reduce the consumer base for the club and the league into the future. The implications of drug control destruction of revenue for international athletics, engulfed in a drug control crisis through 2015 and 2016, remain to be seen. It is therefore pertinent to be aware that drug management introduced to prevent revenue destruction may actually become a form of revenue destruction itself.

Revenue creation

As argued in Chapter 1, there is significant scope for drug management to create revenue for sport. The corollary with revenue destruction is that drug management needs to create more revenue for sport than it costs to implement that drug management.

First, the explicit management of integrity processes appears to create value in sport. Mazanov, Lo Tenero, Connor, and Sharpe (2012) showed that the average share price of Italian Serie A clubs implicated in a referee-fixing scandal increased well above the market trend once the scandal had concluded. While it is impossible to correlate the increase in share price to any single aspect of the scandal or the response to the scandal, integrity management protocols implemented in response to the scandal appear to have contributed to the creation of value in terms of share price. Investors appeared to attribute greater value to sports organisations that engage in explicit integrity management. Translating the notion that consumers like integrity management to drug management, similar increases in value might emerge when a sport introduces drug control. For example, the introduction of anti-doping to mixed martial arts in 2015 (through the International Mixed Martial Arts Federation and Ultimate Fighting Championship) offers an opportunity to assess what effect drug-led integrity management has on broadcast and sponsorship revenues.

Revenue creation may stem from increasing the consumer base. In contrast with revenue destruction via drug management dissuading parents from letting children participate in sport, drug management could also create revenue through giving parents confidence sport provides an appropriate social context for their children. For example, parents may be concerned about the integrity of other activities that are less explicit about managing integrity, and therefore encourage children towards sports participation (cf. Boufous, Finch, & Bauman, 2004). Given the correlation between participation and consumption, this helps grow the next generation of consumers. Effective drug management could also create revenue by enabling people to participate in sport for longer. For example, where an athlete might otherwise have to conclude their active involvement in sport due to ageing, judicious drug control can enable sport to continue drawing on revenue from drug-assisted athletes across their life span (Marcora, 2016). An unexpected (and, at the time of writing, theoretical) form of revenue creation emerges from attracting new consumers dissatisfied with drug control in other market sectors. For example, paralleling concerns around the role of drugs in sport, there are concerns over the role of drugs in performing arts, with claims of drug use to enhance performances among classical musicians (Brantigan, Brantigan, & Joseph, 1982; Kenny, 2011) and dancers (Boardley, Allen, Simmons, & Laws, 2016; Sekulic, Peric, & Rodek, 2010). Consumers exposed to drug use, misuse and abuse in the performing arts may feel that the rules- and values-based expectations have been violated, and seek an alternative that manages integrity (at least with regards to drugs) more explicitly. As a result, drug management can expand revenue creation through the consumer base in both expected and unexpected ways.

Revenue creation can also come in the form of how drug management can contribute to creating new markets. This has already been demonstrated by the growth in sports supplement manufacturing, the development of sports specific drugs and the rise of the sports medicine and sports science industries. It has also been demonstrated through anti-doping introducing an entire industry designed to support the policy, including responding to administrative requirements, researching drug detection technologies and anti-doping education. While this might be thought of as a combination of the 'doping and anti-doping industries' (Fincouer *et al.*, 2015; Mazanov & Connor, 2010), the general point is that drug management has the potential to create revenue by creating new markets.

Drug management could also create revenues by manufacturing scandal. Connor and Mazanov (2010) argue that sports scandal has a remarkable capacity to drive media content. Where sports have a relationship with media outlets (e.g. media companies are owners or part owners of sports), drug scandal creates revenue, especially when the scandals are of sufficient magnitude to compel saturation coverage. For example, if it were inclined, Google may be able to estimate the global impact of the Lance Armstrong case on internet traffic and associated advertising (e.g. news sites, fan sites, web logs and discussion boards).

Combining revenue creation and destruction

As noted at the outset, it is the combination of destruction and creation that determines the revenue implications of drug control for sport. In the case of anti-doping, the aversion of destruction and promotion of creation needs to combine to at least US$500 million to justify the investment. Noting the revenue implications of anti-doping are effectively unknown, the size of global sports revenue suggests that the modest investment in drug control is capable of providing a return on investment.

The discussion around revenue destruction and creation builds on the case for a broader discussion of governance with a more detailed look at the risk management of drug control for sport (see Chapter 8). This includes managing risks that reduce revenue, as well as managing risks that increase revenue.

One way to address revenue risks associated with drug control-led integrity management of sport is careful management of the people who make the decisions. This ranges from the athlete who risks being uncompetitive yet abstains from drugs, to the programme manager who signs a lucrative sponsorship deal with a supplements manufacturer. This raises the question whether sport can manage integrity with regards to drugs with more effective management of people involved in sports production. That is, integrity management through drug control may be well served by hiring people to produce sport able to reflect the rules- and values-based expectations of consumers. Examining how human resource management can drive drug control-led integrity management for sport is therefore warranted (see Chapter 9).

It is also relevant to consider the ways in which sport manages the risks of both the consumption of drugs in sporting contexts and the management of that consumption. A key part of that risk evolves from managing the commercial relationship that arises from the presence of drugs in sport (e.g. e-cigarette sponsorships), captured in this context by marketing. Marketing clearly plays a central role in drug control-led integrity management in sport, ranging from sponsorship to managing scandal to using drug control as a marketing device that deserves deeper consideration (see Chapter 10).

The business of managing drugs in sport

As drugs have formed an increasing part of sports practice, so too has the management of drugs in sport become an increasing part of sports business activity. The collection of business activities associated with drug control-led integrity management indicates the emergence of an entire business within sport to manage drugs. This makes examination of the business of managing drugs in sport central, ranging from conceptual problems such as the implications of drugs in sport for business ethics, to more practical problems associated with enabling people to preserve the integrity of sport.

References

Bennett, G., Ferreira, M., Lee, J., & Polite, F. (2009). The role of involvement in sports and sport spectatorship in sponsor's brand use: The case of Mountain Dew and action sports sponsorship. *Sport Marketing Quarterly, 18*(1), 14–24.

Boardley, I. D., Allen, N., Simmons, A., & Laws, H. (2016). Nutritional, medicinal, and performance enhancing supplementation in dance. *Performance Enhancement and Health, 4*(1–2), 3–11.

Boufous, S., Finch, C., & Bauman, A. (2004). Parental safety concerns – a barrier to sport and physical activity in children? *Australian and New Zealand Journal of Public Health*, *28*(5), 482–486.

Brantigan, C. O., Brantigan, T. A., & Joseph, N. (1982). Effect of beta blockade and beta stimulation on stage fright. *American Journal of Medicine*, *72*(1), 88–94.

Connor, J., & Mazanov, J. (2010). The inevitability of scandal: Lessons for sponsors and administrators. *International Journal of Sports Marketing and Sponsorship*, *11*(3), 212–220.

Donnelly, P. (2015). What if the players controlled the game? Dealing with the consequences of the crisis of governance in sports. *European Journal for Sport and Society*, *12*(1), 11–30.

Evans, D. C., & Evans, G. E. (2014). Stakeholder interests from behind the veil: A Rawlsian approach to ethical corporate governance. *Management and Organizational Studies*, *1*(2), 148–154.

Finocouer, B., van de Ven, K., & Mulrooney, K. (2015). The symbiotic evolution of anti-doping and supply chains of doping substances: How criminal networks may benefit from anti-doping policy. *Trends in Organized Crime*, *18*(3), 229–250.

Foster, G., O'Reilly, N., & Davila, A. (2016). *Sports Business Management: Decision Making Around the Globe*. Abingdon: Routledge.

Gowthorp, L., Greenhow, A., & O'Brien, D. (2016). An interdisciplinary approach in identifying the legitimate regulator of anti-doping in sport: The case of the Australian Football League. *Sport Management Review*, *19*(1), 48–60.

Heneghan, C., Howick, J., O'Neill, B., Gill, P. J., Lasserson, D. S., Cohen, D., *et al.* (2012). The evidence underpinning sports performance products: a systematic assessment. *BMJ Open*, *2*(4), e001702.

Hosseini, J. C., & Brenner, S. N. (1992). The stakeholder theory of the firm: a methodology to generate value matrix weights. *Business Ethics Quarterly*, *2*(2), 99–119.

Kenny, D. (2011). *The Psychology of Music Performance Anxiety*. Oxford, UK: Oxford University Press.

Lippi, G., Sanchis-Gomar, F., & Banfi, G. (2012). Anti-'negative-doping' testing: a new perspective in anti-doping research? *European Journal of Applied Physiology*, *112*(6), 2383–2384.

Maennig, W. (2014). Inefficiency of the anti-doping system: Cost reduction proposals. *Substance Use and Misuse*, *49*(9), 1201–1205.

Marcora, S. (2016). Can doping be a good thing? Using psychoactive drugs to facilitate physical activity behaviour. *Sports Medicine*, *46*(1), 1–5.

Mazanov, J. (2013). *Vale* WADA, *ave* 'World Sports Drug Agency'. *Performance Enhancement and Health*, *2*(2), 80–83.

Mazanov, J. (2014). Drug control in sport: Who and how. In B. Stewart & M. Burke (Eds.). *Drugs and Sport: Writings from the Edge* (pp. 33–71). Melbourne: Dry Ink Press.

Mazanov, J. (2016). Beyond anti-doping and harm minimisation: A stakeholder-corporate social responsibility approach to drug control for sport. *Journal of Medical Ethics*, *42*(4), 220–223.

Mazanov, J., & Connor, J. (2010). Rethinking the management of drugs in sport. *International Journal of Sport Policy*, *2*(1), 49–63.

Mazanov, J., Lo Tenero, G., Connor, J., & Sharpe, K. (2012). Scandal + football = A better share price. *Sport, Business, Management, 2*(2), 92–114.

Miles, S. (2012). Stakeholder: essentially contested or just confused? *Journal of Business Ethics, 108*(3), 285–298.

Outram, S. M., & Stewart, B. (2015). Should nutritional supplements and sports drinks companies sponsor sport? A short review of the ethical concerns. *Journal of Medical Ethics, 41*(6), 447–450.

Paoli, L., & Donati, A. (2014). *The Sports Doping Market*. New York: Springer.

Phillips, R. A. (1997). Stakeholder theory and a principle of fairness. *Business Ethics Quarterly, 7*(1), 51–66.

PWC (2011). Changing the game: Outlook for the global sports market to 2015. Available at: www.pwc.com/gx/en/hospitality-leisure/pdf/changing-the-game-outlook-for-the-global-sports-market-to-2015.pdf (accessed 24 January 2016).

Sekulic, D., Peric, M., & Rodek, J. (2010). Substance use and misuse among professional ballet dancers. *Substance Use and Misuse, 45*(9), 1420–1430.

Solberg, H., Hanstad, D. V., & Thøring, T. (2010). Doping in elite sport – Do the fans care? Public opinion on the consequences of doping scandals. *International Journal of Sports Marketing & Sponsorship, 11*(3), 185–199.

Summers, J., & Johnson, M. (1999). Segmentation of the Australian Sport Market. In A. K. Manrai, & H. L. Meadow (Eds.), *Global Perspectives in Marketing for the 21st Century* (pp. 481–486). Cham, Switzerland: Springer International.

Chapter 6

Business ethics and drug control for sport

The introduction of the distinction between stockholders and stakeholders by corporate social responsibility (CSR) (Carroll, 1991) also informs the distinction between competing definitions of 'rightness' that shape drug control-led integrity management of sport. As sport evolved from amateur enterprise to multinational global mega-events (see Chapter 3), discussion around the ethics of drugs in sport retained a focus on the private interest concerns of amateurism (stockholders) rather than the more public concerns of sport as a modern business (stakeholders). This has seen contemporary debate over drug control for sport focus on the ethics of anti-doping as it pertains to fairness and cheating in competition (e.g. Angelo Corlett, 2013; Bonte, Sterckx, & Pennings, 2014; Morgan, 2006; Wiesing, 2011) or the ethics of anti-doping more broadly (e.g. Loland, 2002; Park, 2005; Tamburrini, 2006; Waddington & Smith, 2009) rather than the ethics of how drug control influences the business of sport (e.g. Carstairs, 2003; Malloy & Zakus, 2002; Schneider & Butcher, 2001). In this sense, while discussion about the ethics of doping in sport is relatively mature, discussion around the business ethics of drug control in sport is yet to reach similar maturity.

The ethical basis to drug control-led integrity management of sport espoused in the anti-doping policy uses a virtues- or values-based approach through the Spirit of Sport statement, as discussed in Chapters 4 and 9. This approach makes a judgement that doping is wrong and that being 'doping free' is right. Drug control-led integrity management has generalised this judgement such that drug consumption in sport is wrong and 'drug-free' sport is right. This judgement is challenged by considering an alternative set of values making a judgement that it is right for stakeholders to prioritise athlete welfare in sport. The challenge from a values-based perspective is then extended by briefly exploring how basic teleological and deontological approaches also challenge the dominant Spirit of Sport-based approach. A consequence of this argument is a need to transcend assumptions of universalism and recognise that the ethics of drug control for sport must address its context within broader society far more explicitly.

As an introduction to how business ethics might inform drug control for sport, an ethically monist approach has been taken. That is, the ethical approaches are considered in isolation from each other to support the point that the Spirit statement represents one of many plausible ways to interpret the role of drugs, drug control and integrity management for sport.

Virtues and the Spirit of Sport

According to de George (2009), the starting point for virtues-based approaches to ethics is making a judgement about the rightness of behaviour. The Aristotelian approach argues the capacity to make a judgement about the rightness of behaviour emerges from hard-won wisdom through experience with both virtues and vices. This wisdom is demonstrated through the intellectual (rational) and moral (proper control of natural inclinations that lead to vice) virtues of an individual that enable them to exist within a society. The patterns of dispositions (character) that enable people to live in society with others then describe the qualities that make a person virtuous. As de George argues, good people are good because they do what they ought within their society. The qualities that make a person virtuous can and should be taught by those who have amassed enough experience (wisdom) to be considered virtuous.

Given the foundations of ancient sport as a religious festival and modern sport as a socialising force (see Chapter 3), it is perhaps no surprise that sport adopted the virtues-based approach to managing drugs by judging doping as a vice to be controlled through intellectual and moral virtue. Those who dope, or are deemed complicit in doping in some way, have failed to control their natural inclinations and compromised the qualities that enable athletes to participate in sports societies. It is hoped that those whose moral virtues need to be developed can be educated to achieve the relevant virtues (Hoberman, 2013). Those who dope are excluded from athletic societies until such time as they gain enough experience to see the wisdom of the judgement against doping and demonstrate the appropriate virtues. That is, sport has made a moral judgement that doping is wrong and that dopers should be punished (O'Leary, 2001, p. 256).

Genesis of the Spirit statement

The virtues which enable the judgement that doping is wrong flow from the 11 values declared as the basis of Olympism that make up the Spirit statement (see Table 6.1). Ritchie (2013) provides an account of the Spirit statement's genesis, which began as part of Canada's response to the crisis arising from the 1988 Seoul Olympics and the ensuing Dubin Inquiry. Dubin argued that sport needed to rediscover ethics and morality in opposition to the obsession with 'winning gold', with values that met the

Table 6.1 Values and drug control for sport: the Spirit of Sport and athlete welfare

	Spirit of Sport (as per the Code)	Athlete welfare (alphabetical order)
Judgement	Drugs are wrong, users punished	Promote athlete welfare
1	Ethics, fair play, honesty	Athlete control
2	Health	Education
3	Excellence in performance	Personal growth
4	Character and education	Sporting capital
5	Fun and joy	Sustainable participation
6	Teamwork	Transparency
7	Dedication and commitment	
8	Respect for rules and laws	
9	Respect for self and other participants	
10	Courage	
11	Community and solidarity	

promotion of mass participation sport as both a public and social good (Ritchie, 2013, p. 197). From this point of view, Dubin argued that drugs should be considered the antithesis of sport, presumably as a symptom of the obsession with winning (noting that treating a symptom can fail to remedy the underlying pathogen). Values such as fairness and the role of sport in socialising citizens ('character-building') were considered more appropriate foundations of sport. The Canadian Centre for Drug Free Sport (later the Canadian Centre for Ethics in Sport) created the Spirit of Sport campaign that began to shape the Spirit values.

Drug scandals arising from the 1998 Tour de France and World Swimming Championships spurred the formation of WADA (see Chapter 3) – with development of the World Anti-Doping Code (the Code) overseen by a five-person Code Project Team (Ritchie, 2013, p. 198). The Canadian values were tested as part of the extensive international consultation that led to the Code, resulting in the values described in the Spirit statement being established as the universal basis for Olympism and the ethical basis for anti-doping. At the time of writing, the Spirit statement had survived all three Code revisions without amendment. The extensive consultation that underpins the Code and its reviews means the Spirit statement could be argued to represent the collective wisdom of sports participants that has led to a 'grounded theory' of the values that underpin Olympism. An alternative view is that the Spirit statement reflects the mental model of what the Code Project Team thought sport ought to be (Mazanov & Huybers, 2016) whose wisdom is presumed inviolable.

Irrespective of whether the Spirit statement reflects the summative view of the many, or the normative view (and vested interest; Carstairs, 2003;

Mazanov, 2014; O'Leary, 2001) of a few, in practice the Spirit statement is treated as the set of values that underpins *all* sport, rather than just Olympism. This ethical hegemony has developed from the Code establishing that any activity which fails to follow Olympism no longer being considered a legitimate sport. For example, Jedlicka (2014) observes that the only way to be considered a legitimate (drug-free) sport is to agree with the values of Olympism. The consequence of this is that the Code and Spirit statement exclude any activity which is outside Olympism, such as professional sports (e.g. darts) (Kornbeck, 2013, p. 316). The ethical hegemony emerges in practice with activities seeking government funding as a sport needing to be Code compliant (as signatories to the International Convention against Doping in Sport). For example, the Fédération Internationale des Echecs (World Chess Federation) adopted the Spirit values, in part, to enable national chess organisations to access government sports-related funding (e.g. Germany and Canada; Golf, 2015). That is, chess was forced to give up its own ethical identity and adopt the values of Olympism, with no regard for whether the values of Olympism were appropriate for chess. The longer this process continues the more likely the values of the Spirit statement will become the universal values of sport simply because it has effectively eliminated any competing values or ethical approaches to sport. It is therefore crucial that the values making up the Spirit statement are well defined and well understood.

Poorly defined and variably understood

As argued in Chapters 4 and 9, ambiguity rather than precision is a feature of the Spirit statement. Some see this as a strength (McNamee, 2012), while others argue that the failure to provide meaningful guidance on the assumed universal values base for sport creates significant problems for management specifically and sport generally (Loland & Hoppeler, 2012; Mazanov & Connor, 2010). Linguistic variation can create difficulties for managers working in cross-cultural contexts (e.g. professional football) trying to explain why athletes should be Code compliant. For example, 'health' has different meanings across languages; meaning 'absence of illness or injury' in English (absence of a negative), but 'fitness' or 'soundness' (υγεία) in Greek (presence of a positive).

Kornbeck (2013) argues that the Spirit values are intentionally biased and imprecise to achieve ideological aims at the expense of operational certainty (p. 316). For example, the ambiguity in the Spirit statement values enables a 'stunning degree of elasticity' for administrators (p. 326). This elasticity emerges within sport through the Spirit statement being used as a catch-all phrase that effectively allows the prohibition of any drug (see Chapter 4). This has led to a Code designed to control one type of drug consumption (doping) ending up controlling drugs that have no implications for sport (e.g. masking agents). Arguments have also been advanced that the catch-all nature of the Spirit statement allows anti-doping agencies to inappropriately govern the private, non-sporting lives of athletes both in terms of autonomy (e.g. restricting non-sport related drug consumption; Waddington, Christiansen, Gleaves, Hoberman, & Møller, 2013) and freedom of movement (e.g. out-of-competition testing) (Stewart & Smith, 2014). The elasticity emerges outside sport with the Australian Government justifying coercive powers that compel citizens (including those with no direct relationship with sport) to give evidence for sports drug investigations deemed to protect the integrity of sport (Alexander, 2014). It seems that the ambiguity in the Spirit statement can be reconstructed to achieve any particular end in pursuit of promoting the anti-doping ideology.

The Spirit statement can also be variably understood. The Spirit statement values can be thought to be presented as a hierarchy, with 'ethics, fair play and honesty' considered the most important value, 'health' the second most important and so on to 'community and solidarity' being considered the least important value. Alternatively, the values could be considered equally important irrespective of position in the notional hierarchy presented in the Code. The former provides clear guidance to managers on how to prioritise the values. Meeting an administrative test based on the latter may make deploying drug control unfeasible. This immediately raises questions about whether the Spirit statement is the universal ethical basis for sport. Empirically, Mazanov and Huybers (2016) demonstrated that Australians produce different hierarchies to those implied by the Code across samples, and that Australians ranked the Spirit values differently across elite and non-elite sporting contexts. Whether other cultures match the Code or Australian hierarchy, or report different hierarchies, remains to be seen.

It is a little surprising that the Spirit statement has received so little attention. First, the survival of the Spirit statement unchanged despite multiple revisions to the Code could be a function of a lack of interest in the Spirit statement by those making submissions to Code Review consultations, or that those responsible for Code revisions take the view that the Spirit statement needs no revision. Second, it is surprising that the academic literature has given so little attention to a values-statement declared as the fundamental basis for a practice that reaches across the global community (McNamee, 2012).

New wisdom on drug control for sport

The claim that the Spirit statement represents values universal to all sport is contestable. By corollary, the justification for anti-doping as the fundamental basis for drug control in sport is also contestable. Indeed, the premise that doping is somehow definitionally wrong has been fiercely debated. It may be appropriate to develop a new judgement on the role of drugs in sport by learning from the experience with the Spirit statement.

The Spirit statement approach to virtues appears to make an assumption that those who have deemed doping immoral for Olympic sport have the wisdom to make the judgement for all sport, all types of drugs and all forms of drug consumption (use, misuse or abuse). That is, there is an assumption that the wisdom received from the five-person Code Project Team and confirmed by the custodians of the Code Review processes is inviolable and immutable over time.

However, the prescribed exclusion of non-Olympic sport creates uncertainty as to whether the wisdom of the Spirit statement extends beyond the bounds of Olympic sport, or takes into account the wisdom of those directly affected by drug control – the athletes (Mazanov, 2014). Equally, given the profound implications for those well outside sport, the interests of those affected indirectly by anti-doping also need to be accounted for. It may be more appropriate to transcend the Olympic stockholder views to introduce the views from different forms of sport and different perspectives (e.g. those outside sport) in coming to a new judgement about the role of drugs in sport.

The exoneration of sporting institutions from responsibility for drug control by individualising the phenomenon is also problematic. This has been expressed in the Code as athletes being objects (done *to* athletes to protect the virtue of sport) rather than subjects of drug control (done *for* athletes upholding the virtue of sport) (Houlihan, 2004; Kreft, 2011). There is an assumption that the inability to control drug vice lies with the individual. This assumption has prevailed even though it was well understood before the first iteration of the Code that the practice of drug behaviour in sport occurs within a complex web of social and institutional structures (e.g. British Medical Association, 2002). A more explicit account of institutional interests in the role of drugs in sport may also contribute towards a new judgement.

A different virtues approach to drug control for sport

A virtues approach to drug control for sport may still be viable by working towards a different judgement about the role of drugs in sport. The policy alternatives in Chapter 4 offer guiding principles that might be used to replace the foundation judgement. For example, a fully prohibitionist approach implies a narrow understanding of naturalness and authenticity in performance as the values. Harm-minimisation places athlete medicalised health (fitness to compete) as the only value of concern to sport. The handicap approach suggests fairness might be the dominant value. Finally, a laissez-faire approach suggests personal freedoms could be the dominant value. These approaches all have the character of stockholders' private interests at the expense of others outside sport who may have a legitimate interest in sport (stakeholders).

One existing approach that may provide a core judgement satisfactory to both stockholders and stakeholders is explicitly accounting for the role of sports as modern businesses, as suggested by Verroken (2001, p. 38). For example, Mendoza (2002) argues that the best ethical defence for drug control in sport rests on community preference. The stakeholder approach to CSR (Mazanov, 2016) may be an appropriate way to guide a virtues approach to drug control for sport. The stakeholder approach argues that those potentially affected by an organisation have a legitimate moral interest in how that organisation conducts itself. This stands in contrast to the Spirit statement, where the interests of administrative convenience appear to have been given priority. Applying the arguments from Chapter 1, the primary judgement concerning the role of drugs in sport is one that addresses survival and profit concerns across stakeholders.

Athlete welfare – the cornerstone of survival and profit

The development of sport as a commodity depends upon being able to attract and retain a sufficient participation base (e.g. athletes and support personnel) to create sports events, whether competitive or recreational. Given athletes are the foundation production unit without whom sport no longer exists, athletes should have the dominant role in making the moral judgement about what role drugs might play in sport (Mazanov, 2014). For example, the moral judgement about the role of drugs in sport may be to promote survival of the participation base by preserving athlete welfare (in terms of physical, psychological and social health) in the interests of protecting and promoting participation (e.g. having fun), thereby driving survival of the sport. That is, the moral judgement is that drugs have a legitimate place in sport to the extent they enable athletes to participate in sport (cf. Marcora, 2016). The corollary is that drugs have no place in sport if they diminish athlete capacity to participate in sport. For example, athletes can decide that doping diminishes sport by forcing people to use drugs when they would otherwise abstain (coercive effects). With this judgement in place, the interests of stakeholders shape the values that drive what is considered a legitimate role for drugs (see Table 6.1).

Stakeholders and survival

To promote survival, the values associated with drug control need to be consistent with attracting new participants and consumers. Parents become critical stakeholders in the survival of a sport. For example, parents may need to feel that their children are entering an appropriate developmental environment that promotes personal growth through sport (see Chapter 5). The values associated with survival then become addressing the role of drugs facilitating personal growth; for example, junior sport may remain focused on drug use that prevents illness and/or injury (promoting participation), while taking the view that unnecessary use, misuse or abuse of drugs (e.g. caffeine or alcohol) diminishes personal growth.

The capacity to deliver sports events, from ad hoc community sports to mega-events (e.g. the Olympics), is usually critically contingent upon volunteers (Cuskelly & Auld, 2012). The donation of time means volunteers have a legitimate moral interest in drug control. Volunteers typically donate their time as an expression of belief in contributing to a worthwhile community activity and the potential for personal growth (including career) (e.g. Hallman & Harms, 2012). In terms of drug control, volunteers could contribute by helping athletes navigate drugs that promote and diminish athlete welfare. In doing so, volunteers can also learn more about the role of drugs in sport and drugs in society that supports making their own informed decisions about drugs. The value implied here is that education about drugs and their role in sport may be appropriate.

Governments are key stakeholders in the survival of sport for a range of political, social and public health reasons (Houlihan, 2002). Governments look to minimise the burdens arising from sports participation (e.g. regulating drugs, injury or drug abuse) while promoting sport for its economic, symbolic, cultural, social, physical and psychological capital building capacity (Stewart & Smith, 2014); that is, sporting capital (see Chapter 1). As a result, the values that governments might impose relate to minimising the burdens of sport and maximising the benefits. The difficulty for governments is ensuring policy coherence and consistency. For example, drugs that enable Masters level athlete participation may be considered consistent with policies aimed at addressing physical activity. Conversely, supplying subsidised drugs to children for the purposes of sports participation may be seen as an inappropriate use of public funds.

Insurance companies may create barriers to sport by adjusting premiums based on the relative risks associated with participating in different sports. For example, athletes using drugs known to reduce the relative risk of chronic illness or injury arising from participation in sport may find it easier (cheaper) to access sport, and therefore improve the chances of a sport achieving sustainable levels of participation. Further, event organisers may find it easier to get insurance if the sport regulates the role of drugs to maximise athlete welfare. This might include the explicit management of alcohol (e.g. no alcohol sponsorship or an alcohol-free event) to minimise alcohol-related harms. This suggests a level of transparency around drug consumption may have some merit.

Stakeholders and profit

For the purposes of this discussion, profit is the point at which third parties introduce capital (e.g. sponsorship) that takes the sport beyond subsistence. This investment establishes the legitimate moral interest in production. However, the primary concern of stakeholders who bring profit to sport is less about production processes and more about consuming the outcome of those production efforts. For example, consuming the outcome of production may see interests in athlete welfare marginalised in pursuit of spectacle. This creates a tension between stakeholders with an interest in the survival of a sport, and stakeholders with an interest in profiting from sport.

'Fans' are the kernel of consumption that translates survival into profit; those people who invest time and money to engage with the outcome of sports production efforts. What fans derive from sport varies from a sense of community fundamental to self- and social identity to an occasional escape from the realities of daily life (e.g. Funk, Beaton, & Alexandris, 2012). This also varies between levels of sport, demonstrated by the values for non-elite sport being constructed differently to elite sport (e.g. Mazanov & Huybers, 2016). Given this variability, to advance the discussion the essence of what fans may value is summarised as a psychological contract with sports that enables access to events for transactional benefits (e.g. investing time in exchange for desired experiences). The interests of fans therefore relate to the outcome rather than the process of sports production. History shows that fans consume sport despite concerns with production processes; for example, fans appear to be willing to consume sport despite evidence of systematic doping (Buechel, Emrich, & Pohlkamp, 2014). Fan interests may be represented by the idea that drugs should promote athlete welfare without transgressing other judgements about the role of drugs in society (e.g. illicit drugs).

Attracting participants and fans makes access to sports events a valuable commodity to advertisers, sponsors and broadcasters. Advertisers and sponsors are looking for exposure and brand association with a sport (see Chapter 10). (Note that this is different to the relationship with an individual athlete, such as Lance Armstrong.) Broadcasters are interested in maximising audiences to on-sell advertising. Drug control may have an impact on mass participation events; for example, anti-doping can limit the potential market for Masters Games participants by denying access to athletes on prohibited drugs for therapeutic reasons (Henning & Dimeo, 2015). Advertisers', sponsors' and broadcasters' interests are best served by drawing as many people to participate in the event as possible. There is also an interest that audiences are at least maintained or grow. Doping has had a modest impact on broadcast audiences in both the Tour de France (Buechel *et al.*, 2014; van Reeth, 2013) and Major League Baseball (average 8 per cent reduction in home game attendance lasting 15 days) (Cisyk & Courty, 2015). However, these changes may be a response to the moral panic constructed around doping (Crichter, 2014; McDermott, 2016) rather than the role of drugs in sport. An athlete welfare approach to drug control may mitigate such effects. Conversely, audiences tend to maximise when celebrity athletes participate in prestigious events that are competitively interesting (Konjer, Meier, & Wedeking, 2015; Rodríguez, Pérez, Puente, & Rodríguez, 2015). As a result, the value at play here may be to allow athlete drug use that enables participation without compromising athlete welfare (e.g. playing on pain killers).

The legal gambling industry (as opposed to illegal gambling and organised crime) takes a legitimate interest in sports production. The interest here is that consumers (gamblers) have access to information to estimate outcomes. The absence of information that impact outcomes distorts estimates, skewing the gamble in favour of some at the expense of many. The principle is that the relativities are understood from the outset; such as gamblers accepting the fixed (usually low) probability of winning associated with a lottery or a specific number on a roulette wheel. Under athlete welfare, athlete privacy (social health) needs to be traded against gambling interests in transparency. For example, it may be inappropriate for gamblers to know that an athlete is being treated for a legitimate medical condition (e.g. depression). The value that might be imposed here is for a limited form of transparency that gives gamblers sufficient information to make assessments about potential performance implications of drugs without compromising athlete welfare (e.g. privacy). For example, information might be given about the drugs used within a sports programme without going into specific details about individual athletes.

The starting point for alternative values

Evaluating how a moral judgement that athlete welfare should be the foundation for drug control might be shaped by stakeholder interests identifies some potential values that contrast with the anti-doping policy. The values are suggested in alphabetical order (see Table 6.1), with no implication for order or relative value. The first value reflects that athletes should have control over what is in the best interests of their welfare. The second is that educating stakeholders about the role of drugs in sport is essential to promote athlete welfare. The third draws on the notion that athlete welfare is best served when drugs enable personal growth, drawing on experiences of the self and others to guide decisions. Sporting capital as a value looks to enable and promote access to the benefits of sport for the individual and society. The fifth value aims to incorporate drugs into sport in such a way that it enables sustainable participation, from teaching adolescents about nutrition to Masters athletes using prescription drugs to enable participation. The final value is transparency in consumption to promote athlete welfare (e.g. detection of misuse or abuse, or drug exploitation).

Virtues and drug control for sport

The Spirit statement represents a strong starting position to debate the virtues of drug control for sport. The Code Project Team is to be commended for reconciling the breadth and depth of sport into such a small set of values. As Mazanov (2016) argues, rather than defending the Spirit statement as the only possible consequence of rational and moral virtue, the Spirit statement needs to be debated and modified as experience with drug control grows. This can be achieved by considering alternatives. The moral judgement that athlete welfare should be the primary concern for sports production offers an alternative and a starting point for debate.

Extending the debate to other ethical perspectives

While the virtues approach has dominated the discussion to this point, there are other standard approaches that merit consideration as potential ethical foundations to drug control for sport. The two discussed here are the teleological and deontological approaches. The starting point for such consideration is to address drug control for sport generally rather than addressing concerns arising from the presumed distortion of outcomes specific to doping (e.g. fairness and naturalness).

Teleology and drug control for sport

Teleological approaches to ethics assess the rightness of a behaviour based on its ends (de George, 2009). The dominant form of teleology is consequentialism, where actions are assessed based on their consequences. While an action itself has no particular moral value, the consequences of that action are assessed in their context as being right or wrong. For example, the assessment might be made on the basis of how many people benefit from a particular action relative to the number of people harmed (utilitarianism). What constitutes a benefit or a harm forms the basis of different approaches, such as hedonistic (pleasure), eudaimonistic (happiness) and ideal utilitarianism (intrinsically valuable human goods). Assessment of benefit and harm is the foundation of teleology, requiring careful, objective and impartial evaluation of consequences.

The teleological issue at stake is whether the consequences of drug control in sport lead to a net benefit or a net harm. For example, a teleological analysis asks whether the presence of a sports specific form of drug control leads to greater benefit than the standard forms of drug control that already exist within a society (cf. Chapter 5). This raises a question about the potential benefits and harms arising from sports specific drug control. Given sports specific drug control brings with it a range of harms both to individuals (e.g. human rights) and societies (e.g. diverting resources), there needs to be a net benefit to both individuals and societies before sport can be considered ethical (cf. Malloy & Zakus, 2002).

Athletes tend to use tobacco and illicit drugs at rates lower than the general population, while misusing or abusing alcohol, nutritional supplements and prescription drugs (doping) at higher rates (Diehl, Thiel, Zipfel, Mayer, & Schneider, 2014; Dunn & Thomas, 2012; Lisha & Sussman, 2010; Martha, Grelot, & Peretti-Watel, 2009; Wichstrøm & Wichstrøm, 2009) (see also Chapter 11). Sport has protective effects against tobacco and illicit drugs without sport specific drug control; the practice of sport creates the consequence of lower consumption. This frees resources to address other issues, which suggests a net benefit without the need for sports specific drug control. Binge alcohol consumption is a known and ongoing problem for both sport and society that has resisted multiple attempts at sports specific and general control. This suggests a net harm, irrespective of whether sports specific alcohol control is in place. As noted in Chapter 2, nutritional supplements are seen as having either positive or neutral health implications, suggesting a net harm from imposing sports specific control. In terms of prescription drugs, the misuse and abuse of prescription drugs with fatal consequences raises a clearly profound harm (Parisotto, 2006). The teleological question is whether drug control for sport would prevent such deaths through controlling misuse or abuse more generally. The inability to develop a reliable epidemiology of misuse or abuse makes it difficult to estimate the extent to which harms can be prevented. Further, some insight into the proportion of athletes who, for example, self-medicate without consequence is needed. It is therefore impossible to declare whether sports specific control of prescription drugs would lead to a net benefit or harm. This brief analysis suggests that there is no particular benefit to introducing sports specific drug control (i.e. the existing drug control for society rather than sport is sufficient), although more evidence is needed to make a judgement on the potential harms associated with prescription drugs.

The next step in a teleological analysis is whether the presence of sports specific drug control creates benefits or harms. Policy evaluation of anti-doping suggests that sports drug control has created little benefit with regards to its stated aims (fairness in competition), but has created significant harms. For example, it is impossible to say whether anti-doping has led to a reduction in any form of drug consumption given little change in the proportion of positive drug tests over time (de Hon, Kuipers, & van Bottenburg, 2015). There is also little evidence that sport is 'fairer', with performances from athletes known to dope statistically indistinct from athletes presumed to be doping free (Hermann & Henneberg, 2015), or has improved the overall health and well-being of athletes (Smith & Stewart, 2008, p. 128). Indeed, the evidence suggests that, despite all the administrative architecture, anti-doping has had little impact on the daily practice of athletes, support personnel or administrators (Chan et al., 2015; Mazanov, Hemphill, Connor, Quirk, & Backhouse, 2015; Houlihan, 2014). Instead, anti-doping appears to have led to a number of consequences that could be considered net harms. Resources have been diverted to establish and sustain anti-doping that may have been diverted to other priorities (e.g. addressing alcohol-related harms in sport). This includes investment in the development of drug tests (that appear to have little impact on fairness outcomes) at the expense of other healthcare priorities (Black, 1996; Kayser, Mauron, & Miah, 2007; Lippi, Franchini, & Guidi, 2008). Sanctions have seen athletes lose their reputation in the community and their livelihood. There are concerns that reporting requirements for out-of-competition testing represent a violation of human rights (Houlihan, 2004; Kreft, 2011). It appears that anti-doping has had little benefit while creating harms. From a teleological point of view, the evidence and argument indicate that the net harm created by the consequences of anti-doping makes it an unethical approach to drug control for sport.

It is acknowledged that the brief review offered is by no means a comprehensive examination of the consequences associated with drug control for sport. A more fine-grained analysis based on a more detailed articulation and assessment of benefits and harms may lead to a different conclusion. This more fine-grained articulation of the consequences of drug control for sport may lead to important insights about the relationship between drugs and sport. For example, applying the teleological lens to the athlete welfare argument asks whether drug control can achieve a net benefit across stakeholders, or leaves some stakeholders so profoundly worse off the athlete welfare approach can also be declared unethical.

Deontology and drug control for sport

Deontological approaches argue that the moral quality of actions can be determined independently of their consequences. As a result, the imperative is that the decision to do right or wrong should be taken without regard for the outcome. The dominant Kantian approach to deontology posits that the process used to rationalise right and wrong can only be imposed on the self by the self (de George, 2009). The process of rationalising right and wrong leads to three tests which define moral action. The first of these is that the action must be consistently universal; that is, rationally follow a rule that can be applied across actors in a consistent way. The second is that the action treats others with respect and dignity. The third test asks whether the action maintains the autonomy of rational beings (self-determination). Moral action passes all three tests; failing any element means the action is immoral.

In terms of consistency, game-theoretic analysis indicates that some athletes always end up doping (see Chapter 8). While similar analysis for other types of drugs is missing, the evidence suggests that the majority of athletes end up consuming some combination of licit drugs, supplements, over-the-counter drugs and prescription drugs as part of their sporting practice (e.g. Hoyte, Albert, & Heard, 2013; Sato *et al.*, 2015; Tscholl, Vaso, Weber, & Dvorak, 2015). To prevent athletes from consuming drugs would be to prevent sport. This suggests a rule where athletes are able to consume drugs is more likely to be consistently universal.

Athlete drug consumption must occur on the basis of dignity and respect for others, across competitors to support personnel to managers to broadcasters. For example, athletes need to respect the basis upon which other athletes choose to compete. Given the result that drug consumption appears to have little impact on performance (Hermann & Henneberg, 2015), there appear to be no grounds for abstinent athletes to refuse to compete against athletes who choose to consume; of course, they are free to do so if they choose. By comparison, drug consumption which impugns the experience of sport for others is unsustainable. For example, the athlete who attacks competitors in the midst of an amphetamine-induced psychotic break clearly impugns the experience of sport for others. This may also include transgressing boundaries of socially acceptable behaviour in relation to drug control (e.g. drunken violence). This indicates that drugs should be controlled based on their potential to diminish the experience of sport among others.

The third test asks that drug control be something that people elect to follow as a consequence of rational deliberation rather than something that people are forced to conform or comply with. For example, athletes support the principles of drug control in sport, but appear to have highly variable views about the mechanisms used to compel compliance with the Code. Some athletes take the view that drug control measures should become more restrictive and punitive (Breivik, Hanstad, & Loland, 2009), whereas others appear to tolerate drug control as a 'necessary evil' of participating in sport (Overbye & Wagner, 2014). This suggests that people are willing to follow drug control for sport, although an alternative to anti-doping might be more widely accepted. For example, athlete support personnel appear willing to help athletes navigate the role of drugs in their sporting practice, especially with regards to misuse or abuse of drugs (Mazanov *et al.*, 2015).

As with the analysis of the teleological approach, the analysis using the three tests of the deontological approach is neither comprehensive nor complete. For example, the discussion omits considerations of duties, rights and justice (de George, 2009). While holding drug control for sport apart from its consequences suggests that drug control is a necessary and acceptable part of sport, exactly what constitutes a failure to respect others can be constructed very differently to the interpretation offered. In realising the aim to provide another alternative to the virtues approach, it seems that there is a viable argument that drug control is something worth investing in. What form drug control might take is predicated on enabling athletes to use drugs, and to do so with regard to the effects that use has on others involved in sport.

Kick starting the business ethics of drug control for sport

The hegemonic nature of anti-doping may see it become the only approach to drug control, irrespective of whether it addresses the implications of integrity management arising from other forms of drug consumption. A much stronger debate about the ethics of drug control for sport, and especially the Spirit statement, is needed to avoid ethical monism taking root. While the approach taken for this chapter was to present different ethical perspectives in isolation, the debate needs to be ethically pluralist to develop a richer justification for drug control.

Part of this debate needs to account for the ethical implications of how drugs moderate or mediate trust that the rules- and values-based expectations in production have been met. These expectations appear to vary significantly across drug types. Part of the problem may lie in the attempt to establish the universal values from the perspective of sport, rather than taking into account interests outside sport. The ethical justification of drug control for sport must account for the broader social context. If sport is to engage in meaningful drug control-led integrity management, it may need to consider what integrity in sport means to stakeholders outside sport. Doing so may yield a defensible basis to the way in which stakeholder interests are prioritised (see Chapter 5).

More generally, the discussion of sports drug control using a business ethics lens indicates managers need to be aware that the integrity of an administrative system is different to integrity management. Unfortunately, sport appears to have created its universal values to resolve administrative rather than integrity concerns. Instead, attempts to manage integrity need to have a deeper understanding of what integrity means both within and between stakeholders. This understanding then enables decisions about acceptable and unacceptable violations of trust across stakeholders.

References

Alexander, B. R. (2014). War on drugs redux: Welcome to the war on doping in sports. *Substance Use and Misuse, 49*(9), 1190–1193.

Angelo Corlett, J. (2013). Doping: Just do it? *Sport, Ethics and Philosophy, 7*(4), 430–449.

Black, T. (1996). Does the ban on drugs in sport improve societal welfare? *International Review for the Sociology of Sport, 31*(4), 367–381.

Bonte, P., Sterckx, S., & Pennings, G. (2014). May the blessed man win: a critique of the categorical preference for natural talent over doping as proper origins of athletic ability. *The Journal of Medicine and Philosophy, 39*(4), 368–386.

Breivik, G., Hanstad, D. V., & Loland, S. (2009). Attitudes towards use of performance-enhancing substances and body modification techniques. A comparison between elite athletes and the general population. *Sport in Society, 12*(6), 737–754.

British Medical Association (2002). *Drugs in Sport: The Pressure to Perform*. London: BMJ Publishing Group.

Buechel, B., Emrich, E., & Pohlkamp, S. (2014). Nobody's innocent: The role of customers in the doping dilemma. *Journal of Sports Economics*, DOI: 10.1177/1527002514551475

Carroll, A. B. (1991). The pyramid of corporate social responsibility: Toward the moral management of organizational stakeholders. *Business Horizons, 34*(4), 39–48.

Carstairs, C. (2003). The wide world of doping: drug scandals, natural bodies, and the business of sports entertainment. *Addiction Research and Theory, 11*(4), 263–281.

Chan, D. K., Donovan, R. J., Lentillon-Kaestner, V., Hardcastle, S. J., Dimmock, J. A., Keatley, D. A., *et al.* (2015). Young athletes' awareness and monitoring of anti-doping in daily life: Does motivation matter? *Scandinavian Journal of Medicine and Science in Sports, 25*(6), e655-e663.

Cisyk, J., & Courty, P. (2015). Do fans care about compliance to doping regulations in sports? The impact of PED suspension in baseball. *Journal of Sports Economics*, DOI: 10.1177/1527002515587441

Crichter, C. (2014). New perspectives on anti-doping policy: From moral panic to moral regulation. *International Journal of Sport Policy and Politics, 6*(2), 153–169.

Cuskelly, G., & Auld, C. (2012). Managing sport volunteers. In L. Trenberth, & D. Hassan (Eds.), *Managing Sport Business: An Introduction* (pp. 247–263). Abingdon: Routledge.

de George, R. T. (2009). *Business Ethics (7th Ed.)*. Upper Saddle River, NJ: Pearson-Prentice Hall.

de Hon, O., Kuipers, H., & van Bottenburg, M. (2015). Prevalence of doping use in elite sports: a review of numbers and methods. *Sports Medicine, 45*(1), 57–69.

Diehl, K., Thiel, A., Zipfel, S., Mayer, J., & Schneider, S. (2014). Substance use among elite adolescent athletes: Findings from the GOAL Study. *Scandinavian Journal of Medicine & Science in Sports, 24*(1), 250–258.

Dunn, M., & Thomas, J. O. (2012). A risk profile of elite Australian athletes who use illicit drugs. *Addictive Behaviors, 37*(1), 144–147.

Funk, D. C., Beaton, A., & Alexandris, K. (2012). Sport consumer motivation: Autonomy and control orientations that regulate fan behaviours. *Sport Management Review*, 15(3), 355–367.

Golf, S. (2015). Doping for chess performance. *Journal of Sports Medicine and Doping Studies*, 5(3).

Hallmann, K., & Harms, G. (2012). Determinants of volunteer motivation and their impact on future voluntary engagement: A comparison of volunteer's motivation at sport events in equestrian and handball. *International Journal of Event and Festival Management*, 3(3), 272–291.

Henning, A. D., & Dimeo, P. (2015). Questions of fairness and anti-doping in US cycling: The contrasting experiences of professionals and amateurs. *Drugs: Education, Prevention and Policy*, 22(5), 400–409.

Hermann, A., & Henneberg, M. (2015). Long term effects of doping in sporting records: 1886–2012. *Journal of Human Sport and Exercise*, 9(3), 727–743.

Hoberman, J. (2013). How much do we (really) know about anti-doping education? *Performance Enhancement and Health*, 2(4), 137–143.

Houlihan, B. (2002). *Dying to Win* (2nd Ed). Strasbourg: Council of Europe Publishing.

Houlihan, B. (2004). Civil rights, doping control and the world anti-doping code. *Sport in Society*, 7(3), 420–437.

Houlihan, B. (2014). Achieving compliance in international anti-doping policy: An analysis of the 2009 World Anti-Doping Code. *Sport Management Review*, 17(3), 265–276.

Hoyte, C. O., Albert, D., & Heard, K. J. (2013). The use of energy drinks, dietary supplements, and prescription medications by United States college students to enhance athletic performance. *Journal of Community Health*, 38(3), 575–580.

Jedlicka, S. (2014). The normative discourse of anti-doping policy. *International Journal of Sport Policy and Politics*, 6(3), 429–442.

Kayser, B., Mauron, A., & Miah, A. (2007). Current anti-doping policy: a critical appraisal. *BMC Medical Ethics*, 8(2).

Konjer, M., Meier, H. E., & Wedeking, K. (2015). Consumer demand for telecasts of tennis matches in Germany. *Journal of Sports Economics*, DOI: 10.1177/1527002515577882

Kornbeck, J. (2013). The naked spirit of sport: A framework for revisiting the system of bans and justifications in the world anti-doping code. *Sport, Ethics and Philosophy*, 7(3), 313–330.

Kreft, L. (2011). Elite sportspersons and commodity control: anti-doping as quality assurance. *International Journal of Sport Policy and Politics*, 3(2), 151–161.

Lippi, G., Franchini, M., & Guidi, G. C. (2008). Doping in competition or doping in sport? *British Medical Bulletin*, 86(1), 95–107.

Lisha, N. E., & Sussman, S. (2010). Relationship of high school and college sports participation with alcohol, tobacco, and illicit drug use: A review. *Addictive Behaviors*, 35(5), 399–407.

Loland, S. (2002). *Fair Play in Sport Competitions. A Moral Norm System*. London: Routledge.

Loland, S., & Hoppeler, H. (2012). Justifying anti-doping: The fair opportunity principle and the biology of performance enhancement. *European Journal of Sport Science*, 12(4), 347–353.

Malloy, D. C., & Zakus, D. H. (2002). Ethics of drug testing in sport – an invasion of privacy justified? *Sport, Education and Society*, 7(2), 203–218.

Marcora, S. (2016). Can doping be a good thing? Using psychoactive drugs to facilitate physical activity behaviour. *Sports Medicine*, 46(1), 1–5.

Martha, C., Grelot, L., & Peretti-Watel, P. (2009). Participants' sports characteristics related to heavy episodic drinking among French students. *International Journal of Drug Policy*, 20(2), 152–160.

Mazanov, J. (2014). Drug control in sport: Who and how. In B. Stewart, & M. Burke (Eds.), *Drugs and Sport: Writings from the Edge* (pp. 33–71). Melbourne, Australia: Dry Ink Press.

Mazanov, J. (2016). Beyond anti-doping and harm minimisation: a stakeholder-corporate social responsibility approach to drug control for sport. *Journal of Medical Ethics*, 42(4), 220–223.

Mazanov, J., & Connor, J. (2010). Rethinking the management of drugs in sport. *International Journal of Sport Policy*, 2(1), 49–63.

Mazanov, J., & Huybers, T. (2016). Societal and athletes' perspectives on doping use in sport: The Spirit of Sport. In V. Barkoukis, L. Lazarus, & H. Tsorbatzoudis (Eds.), *The Psychology of Doping in Sport* (pp. 140–150). Abingdon: Routledge.

Mazanov, J., Hemphill, D., Connor, J., Quirk, F., & Backhouse, S. H. (2015). Australian athlete support personnel lived experience of anti-doping. *Sport Management Review*, 18(2), 218–230.

McDermott, V. (2016). *The War on Drugs in Sport: Moral Panics and Organizational Legitimacy*. Abingdon: Routledge.

McNamee, M. J. (2012). The spirit of sport and the medicalisation of anti-doping: Empirical and normative ethics. *Asian Bioethics Review*, 4(4), 374–392.

Mendoza, J. (2002). The War on Drugs in Sport: A perspective from the front-line. *Clinical Journal of Sport Medicine*, 12(4), 254–258.

Morgan, W. J. (2006). Fair is fair, or is it? A moral consideration of the doping wars in American sport. *Sport in Society*, 9(2), 177–198.

O'Leary, J. (2001). Doping solutions and the problem with 'problems'. In J. O'Leary (Ed.), *Drugs and Doping in Sport: Sociolegal Perspectives* (pp. 255–267). London: Cavendish Publishing.

Overbye, M., & Wagner, U. (2014). Experiences, attitudes and trust: An inquiry into elite athletes' perception of the whereabouts reporting system. *International Journal of Sport Policy and Politics*, 6(3), 407–428.

Parisotto, R. (2006). *Blood sports: the inside dope on drugs in sport*. Prahran, Australia: Hardie Grant.

Park, J. K. (2005). Governing doped bodies: The world anti-doping agency and the global culture of surveillance. *Cultural Studies ↔ Critical Methodologies*, 5(2), 174–188.

Ritchie, I. (2013). The construction of a policy: The World Anti-Doping Code's 'spirit of sport' clause. *Performance Enhancement and Health*, 2(4), 194–200.

Rodríguez, C., Pérez, L., Puente, V., & Rodríguez, P. (2015). The determinants of television audience for professional cycling: The case of Spain. *Journal of Sports Economics*, 16(1), 26–58.

Sato, A., Kamei, A., Kamihigashi, E., Dohi, M., Akama, T., & Kawahara, T. (2015). Use of supplements by Japanese elite athletes for the 2012 Olympic Games in London. *Clinical Journal of Sport Medicine*, 25(3), 260–269.

Schneider, A. J., & Butcher, R. B. (2001). An ethical analysis of drug testing. In W. Wilson, & E. Derse (Eds.), *Doping in Elite Sport: The Politics of Drugs in the Olympic Movement* (pp. 129–152). Champaign, IL: Human Kinetics.

Smith, A., & Stewart, B. (2008). Drug policy in sport: hidden assumptions and inherent contradictions. *Drug and Alcohol Review*, 27(2), 123–129.

Stewart. B., & Smith, A. (2014). *Rethinking Drugs in Sport*. Routledge: UK.

Tamburrini, C. (2006). Are doping sanctions justified? A moral relativistic view. *Sport in Society*, 9(2), 199–211.

Tscholl, P. M., Vaso, M., Weber, A., & Dvorak, J. (2015). High prevalence of medication use in professional football tournaments including the World Cups between 2002 and 2014: A narrative review with a focus on NSAIDs. *British Journal of Sports Medicine*, 49(9), 580–582.

Van Reeth, D. (2013). TV demand for the Tour de France: The importance of stage characteristics versus outcome uncertainty, patriotism, and doping. *International Journal of Sport Finance*, 8(1), 39–60.

Verroken, M. (2001). A time for re-evaluation: The challenge to an athlete's reputation. In J. O'Leary (Ed.), *Drugs and Doping in Sport: Sociolegal Perspectives* (pp. 31–38). Cavendish Publishing: UK.

Waddington, I., & Smith, A. (2009). *An Introduction to Drugs in Sport: Addicted to Winning?* Abingdon: Routledge.

Waddington, I., Christiansen, A. V., Gleaves, J., Hoberman, J., & Møller, V. (2013). Recreational drug use and sport: Time for a WADA rethink? *Performance Enhancement and Health*, 2(2), 41–47.

Wichstrøm, T., & Wichstrøm, L. (2009). Does sports participation during adolescence prevent later alcohol, tobacco and cannabis use? *Addiction*, 104(1), 138–149.

Wiesing, U. (2011). Should performance-enhancing drugs in sport be legalized under medical supervision? *Sports Medicine*, 41(2), 167–176.

Chapter 7

Governance of drugs in sport

The concept of governance is a variably understood and contested term (Geeraert, Alm, & Groll, 2014; MacNamee & Fleming, 2007, p. 427). In the context of corporate social responsibility (CSR) and integrity management, governance aims to promote trust relationships both within and between producers and consumers. Unfortunately, trust relationships in sport have been muddied by the difficult and painful transition from the 'kitchen cabinet' approach to governance of amateur sport to the scrutiny imposed by corporate governance demanded of globalised multinational professional sporting institutions (Donnelly, 2015). Ongoing revelations of corruption (e.g. bribery of officials) to poor governance practices (e.g. accountability and transparency) (Rowbottom, 2013) have earned sport an unenviable reputation.

Historically, the experiences of sports governance in terms of tobacco and alcohol control might be considered a bellwether for the development of a coherent governance of drugs in sport (see Chapter 3). However, the governance of drugs in sport broadly remains fractured, drawing on a range of external bodies. From a governance point of view, the policy coherence offered by anti-doping makes it an attractive foundation to manage the integrity implications of all drugs integral to sport. As a result, this chapter focuses on the governance of anti-doping.

The lead-up to the founding of the World Anti-Doping Agency (WADA) saw intense interest in governance arising from failures across market sectors (e.g. Enron, Worldcom and Tyco) and in the sports sector specifically (e.g. structural reform of the International Olympic Committee; IOC) (MacAloon, 2011). This environment should have seen anti-doping emerge as an exemplar of otherwise elusive 'good governance'. The examination of sports drug control governance indicates that while anti-doping demonstrates some success in relation to systemic governance, there is some way to go before achieving similar success in organisational governance. The governance of drugs in sport shows potential, but 'good governance' remains elusive.

The study of governance draws on a wide-ranging body of theory that overlaps with CSR (e.g. stakeholder theory). Noting the breadth of theory, the approach taken here uses the distinction offered by Ferkins and Van Bottenburg (2013, p. 117), namely the division of governance as the rules governing interactions between institutions (governance between organisations or systemic governance) from the 'what boards do' approach (governance of organisations or organisational governance).

Systemic governance of anti-doping

The strength of anti-doping's systemic governance is premised on policy harmonisation, which has enabled the development of coherent and consistent systemic governance that draws institutions into drug control. The effect is mutually reinforcing systemic governance mechanisms that facilitate institutional interaction for those who take part in the anti-doping network. The system represents 'all but good governance', with anti-doping needing to resolve the ongoing challenge for sport to redress the imbalance towards institutional self-interest at the expense of individual interests (e.g. athletes and support personnel).

The foundation to anti-doping governance

Part 3 of the World Anti-Doping Code (the Code) sets out mutually reinforcing governance principles aimed at achieving policy harmonisation. These principles establish Code compliance as the key criterion to be considered a legitimate sports participant, and that WADA is the final arbiter of whether an institution is compliant (Jedlicka, 2014). Code compliance is given value by making access to the Olympics contingent upon Code compliance. There is a prevailing assumption that the benefits of being able to access Olympic events outweigh the marginal costs of compliance, which sees institutions readily comply. For example, governments willingly create systemic governance structures that promote Code compliance (e.g. setting up anti-doping organisations and regulating non Olympic sports) rather than risk losing tangible (e.g. monetary and structural) and intangible (e.g. national pride) benefits from citizens accessing Olympic events. This mechanism could be used to promote any of the policies outlined in Chapter 4, with the exception of the laissez-faire approach.

Alternatively, an activity seeking legitimation as an international sport can do so by becoming Code compliant, as occurred with chess (see Chapter 6). Like governments, international sports bear the cost of establishing administrative bodies (e.g. specific anti-doping offices) and access the potential to be considered an Olympic event (e.g. raising profile). This approach draws sports into systemic governance of drug control. An overlooked benefit is that compliance eliminates some administrative burdens when seeking government support, such as permission to hold an event. That is, policy harmonisation drives the establishment of a common set of policies and procedures that creates the conditions for administratively efficient institutional interactions (or, depending on the point of view, potentially less burdensome). For example, Code compliance symbolises an institution has adopted standardised administrative processes that can be used as a line of communication between organisations (e.g. contacting the anti-doping office).

Global and European conventions

The systemic governance foundations to anti-doping make agreeing to comply with international conventions a trivial step. Two international conventions govern drug control for sport; the UNESCO International Convention against Doping in Sport and the Council of Europe's (CoE) Anti-Doping Convention. Despite asserting that such drug control is essential to preserve the health of both athletes and sport, none of these documents refer to other drugs that also have health implications (e.g. alcohol and tobacco). This may be intentional, noting that other international conventions and treaties relate to other drugs (e.g. the United Nations Convention Against Illicit Traffic in Narcotic Drugs and Psychotropic Substances and the World Health Organisation Framework Convention on Tobacco Control). The only other form of drugs discussed in these conventions is the UNESCO Convention reference to encouraging the supplement industry to engage in 'best practice'. What that means or how it is monitored is unspecified.

The principles of systemic governance are set out in these conventions, emphasising the need to co-operate internationally and co-ordinate domestically in pursuit of policy harmonisation. Notably, all the documents establish education and research as central to the anti-doping policy. This is presumably premised on the assumption that the rightness of anti-doping will become apparent with sufficient education and experience, and that additional research only reinforces the rightness of the approach (see Møller, 2014; and Chapter 6).

The documents also establish monitoring groups to make decisions on the progress relative to the aims. These monitoring groups effectively represent the accountability and transparency mechanism for the international sports drug control system. This represents a potential weak point in the governance of drug control for sport, with sports governance generally being criticised for making it difficult to find 'published and independently audited detailed accounts of income and expenditure' (Donnelly, 2015, p. 21). While the mechanism is in place, it seems that governance of drug control for sport could be more critical and aggressive with regards to accountability and transparency at the international level (a recommendation of the Independent Commission investigating doping in athletics; see below).

The governance mechanisms make no comment on what happens if the monitoring groups decide anti-doping activity has failed to meet the aims of the conventions. What may happen varies across the documents as a function of their respective histories. The CoE Convention was first ratified in 1989, well before WADA was established. This saw the CoE Convention establish anti-doping through the auspices of international sports organisations. In theory, CoE signatories could abandon the World Anti-Doping Code if they felt it no longer met the aims of the Convention or had been superseded by a better approach to drug control. This allows the CoE a degree of independence.

By comparison, the UNESCO Convention, ratified in 2005, integrates the Code and WADA as a privileged focus for governance of funding (e.g. monitoring contributions), co-operation (e.g. policy models) and advice (e.g. expertise). Unlike the CoE, signatories to the UNESCO Convention have agreed to follow the WADA model. For example, the UNESCO Convention establishes that WADA services should be used to the fullest extent possible. This creates a potential conflict of interest where WADA pursues its legitimate agenda of promoting anti-doping even though it may have failed as a policy or be superseded by a better approach. It is at this point that legitimate institutional self-interest may lead to a governance failure.

Resourcing

Drug control for sport through anti-doping is resourced in two main ways. As noted in Chapter 3, WADA is jointly funded by the IOC and a coalition of governments who have signed the UNESCO Convention. This forces WADA to consider the interests of sport (assuming that IOC interests are representative of all sport, an assumption which is strongly contested; see Donnelly, 2015, p. 20, and Chapter 6) and the public interest when it comes to making decisions about drug control for sport. Of course, the check and balance is critically reliant upon the investment in accountability by those charged with monitoring its activities. That is, the extent to which the agent (in this case WADA) is held to account by the principals (in this case the IOC and coalition of governments).

Top-down governance

The systemic governance mechanisms of the Code and the conventions cascade compliance throughout sports hierarchies (e.g. Kustec Lipicer, & McArdle, 2014; Miller, 2011). For example, Code compliance for both governments and international sports organisations is contingent upon national sports organisations. These flow down through institutions and organisations until the individual is reached. The individual complies with the Code by signing either a contract or a membership statement. From a systemic governance point of view, the cascading compliance is an expression of policy harmonisation where the intentions of the Code are the same no matter where or when sport is practised. This is an impressive feat of administration given the extant difficulties of achieving policy coherence across institutions (Althaus, Bridgman, & Davis, 2013).

Drug control processes

Experience has driven the development of sophisticated governance processes for drug control. Historically, the first major challenge was establishing a robust drug testing protocol. The systemic governance that co-ordinates several institutions in drug testing athletes has been the result of learning what athletes would do to submit clean samples (e.g. prosthetic urethra or anal inserts) through to extensive legal challenges about every element in the chain of custody for drug samples. An integral part of this process has been the development of a system to manage laboratory accreditation (Catlin, Fitch, & Ljungqvist, 2008). Regular audit of laboratory practices enables a level of control and confidence that drug tests meet or exceed standards set by WADA. The system is also flexible enough to accommodate the emergence of new detection technologies, such as the biological passport, which infers drug use by making comparisons across multiple rather than single tests (Sottas & Vernec, 2012).

Experience quickly demonstrated athletes could use drugs in training without testing positive in competition, leading to the development of a remarkable system that allows athletes to be tested at any time. The centralised administration of out-of-competition testing and results management by WADA is given form through the Anti-Doping Administration and Management System (ADAMS), providing an internationally accessible platform to manage anti-doping obligations. It is an indication of the strength of the system that athletes submit to an administrative system (Overbye, 2016; Overbye & Wagner, 2014) that gives anti-doping a level of control over athletes usually reserved for high-risk criminals on parole (Waddington, 2010). For example, athletes must report when and where they will available for testing every day three months in advance. Failure to report availability in advance, or being unavailable at a nominated time and place triggers sanctions. From a systemic governance point of view, this enables tracking of anti-doping administration to, among other management activities, enable efficient and effective reporting and responding.

Dispute resolution

The Code uses the Court of Arbitration for Sport as the appeal mechanism to act as a check and balance and to develop the *lex sportiva*. Sovereign courts can be understandably reluctant to act as an independent review for international sport given complications of jurisdiction. For example, it was found that an Ohio court had no jurisdiction to hear a matter brought by a United States athlete in dispute with a London-based international sports federation about a sample collected in Monaco and tested in France (see Mitten & Opie, 2010). Jurisdictional issues were resolved by forming an arbitration body that heard matters where both parties agreed to abide by the outcomes of tribunal deliberations. While the Court of Arbitration for Sport was troubled by questions over its close relationship with the IOC, a Swiss Federal Court declared it the 'true Supreme Court of international sport' in 2003 (Reilly, 2012). As a result, the Court of Arbitration for Sport has enjoyed a strong reputation as a robust and independent review of drug control matters for sport (although, see below for an alternative view).

Interactions with the pharmaceutical industry

In the same way that governments and sports are drawn into the systemic governance of drug control, systemic governance extends to interactions with private organisations that have an interest in sport. For example, there has been a concerted effort to develop formalised relationships with the pharmaceutical industry (Rabin, 2011), and calls to formalise governance for clinical trials of drugs with potential implications for sport (Camporesi & McNamee, 2014). This has potential positive impacts for pharmaceutical companies looking to associate their brand with sports integrity, penetrate the sports market more generally, or avoid brands being linked with doping scandals (Rabin, 2011). See Chapter 8 for a discussion on risk management of the relationship with the pharmaceutical industry.

Critiques of systemic governance

The strongest critique arising from the systemic governance of anti-doping is that institutional welfare is prioritised over the welfare of individuals. One expression of preserving institutional integrity at the expense of individual integrity can be observed in the harms to the right to privacy, autonomy, self-determination and freedom of movement arising from the surveillance systems giving effect to out-of-competition testing (Houlihan, 2004; Malloy & Zakus, 2002; MacGregor, Griffith, Ruggiu, & McNamee, 2013; Warren, Palmer, & Whelan, 2014). The approach to out-of-competition testing taken by the Code implies that human rights may have been compromised for administrative convenience. The consequence of this approach is that athletes and support personnel become an object to be controlled within a policy looking to preserve institutional integrity rather than describing a process that promotes the integrity of individuals who fall under the policy (Houlihan, 2004; Kreft, 2011). Unfortunately, prioritising institutional interests this way is common in sports governance (Bennett, 2013; Donnelly, 2015).

Further expression can be seen in the codified nature of individualised sanctions in the Code, and the absence of institutional sanctions for governance violations (such as fining sponsors or governments) (see Camporesi & Knuckles, 2014). While the sanctions levelled against the Russian Athletics Federation emerged from doping, the governance mechanism arose from membership with the International Association of Athletics Foundations (IAAF) rather than the Code. The consequence of codifying individuals this way sees athletes at risk of losing control over their own bodies (Henne, 2015; Magdalinski, 2009; Park, 2005), which seems inconsistent with the tenets of 'good governance' and CSR.

Advances in thinking on governance (e.g. CSR) means these issues are by no means insurmountable. The growing interest in the democratisation of sport (e.g. Donnelly, 2015; Geeraert et al., 2014; Parks, 2013) indicates that a more liberal approach to systemic governance would be an appropriate and achievable response. For example, the monitoring groups could conduct their own audits of drug control in specific countries or sports rather than relying on WADA. Another approach might be to diversify the number of principals with an interest in drug control, such as allowing other institutions to contribute to the funding model for WADA (e.g. non-Olympic sports and athlete unions; cf. Kornbeck, 2013; Mazanov, 2014). This may increase the level of scrutiny applied among monitoring groups.

'Good' systemic governance, but ...

The strength of the systems used to govern anti-doping is demonstrated by the breadth of compliance; the majority of nations and sports are signatories to the conventions (Houlihan, 2014). The established mechanisms govern the relationships between institutions, and potentially provide an administrative lingua franca for sport. The systemic governance is held back from being considered 'good governance' by the rather significant implications of the tendency for sports governance to prioritise institutional interests at the expense of individual interests. From an integrity management point of view, systemic integrity may engender institutional trust relationships among sports producers but could potentially threaten the trust sports consumers have in those institutions.

The discussion of anti-doping's systemic governance leads to one particularly valuable insight; that the systems introduced to govern anti-doping could be leveraged to give effect to any sports drug control policy. Should anti-doping be superseded, the systemic governance mechanisms could be adapted to reflect the new policy rather than replace it, leveraging the investment in policy harmonisation for anti-doping. For example, the systems that govern drug testing could be adapted from anti-doping to harm-minimisation in a relatively straightforward manner. This possibility is explored further in Chapter 12.

Organisational governance of anti-doping

While the systemic governance of drug control for sport may be effective independent of the policy, organisational governance is more problematic. For example, while systemic governance has achieved breadth of compliance, there has been little success in terms of depth of compliance where anti-doping shapes individual practice (Houlihan, 2014). This is demonstrated in two ways. The first examines the composition of boards with regards to both conflict of interest and appointment (knowledge and athlete boards). The second looks to the role of boards in overseeing drug control in their sports organisation, drawing on two Australian cases. The first demonstrates how the focus on systemic governance of drug control failed to promote good organisational governance practices, resulting in a compliance approach to drug control. The second demonstrates internal governance failure with a board failing to exercise strategic control over the sports department in the club. At the time of writing, a third case emerged when the Independent Commission report into doping in the IAAF was released, which surprisingly drew on similar themes. These failures suggest that while systemic governance of drug control may be relatively mature, organisational governance practices are in need of further attention.

Board composition and drug control

The importance of the board in sports governance has been expanding with the corporatisation of sport. The traditional hierarchical apprenticeship models of the past (Geeraert et al., 2014) are shifting in response to increasing demands to become the strategic leaders of sport (e.g. Ferkins & Shilbury, 2015). This makes board appointments a crucial aspect of organisational governance, with evidence that a mix of experience and skills is needed on sports boards (Ferkins & Shilbury, 2012). Unfortunately, systemic governance is undermined by organisational governance through the preference for undemocratic board appointments (Geeraert et al., 2014) that appear to advance private political interests of elite administrators rather than the interests of sports organisations or those who participate in sport (Donnelly, 2015). This raises two difficult challenges for organisational governance of drug control for sport. The first is independence of boards and conflict of interest. The second refers back to democratisation issues in terms of representation.

Independence and conflict of interest

While the systemic governance protocols go to great lengths to demonstrate independence using board structures, the restrictions on who can be appointed to a board with responsibility for drug control keeps the organisational governance in check. An example of this emerges from the WADA Boards structures. Appointments to the Foundation Board (responsible for final decisions) and Executive Board are divided between IOC members and member governments (usually Ministers for Sport). The notable exclusion from these boards is non-Olympic sports, compelled to comply with the Code through systemic governance mechanisms.

Many Olympic Board appointments to WADA have multiple roles as elite administrators of international sports, which raise questions about conflicts of interest among Board members. While it makes good sense to have those leading international sport as part of drug control boards, the point here is to recognise the competing interests and their potential to compromise drug control-led integrity management. For example, Pat McQuaid was President of the Union Cycliste Internationale (UCI) 2005–2013 while also an IOC member 2010–2013 and a member of the WADA Foundation (2009–2012) and Executive Committees (2012). It is unclear exactly which set of interests influenced decision making across contexts. The interests of the UCI relative to ongoing doping scandals may have taken precedence over acting in the best interests of the Olympic movement or WADA. Conversely, the UCI may have managed drug control in their sport very differently if the conflicting interests with the Olympic movement or WADA at the board level never existed (Mazanov, 2014). A similar observation may be made about the level of independence in the Independent Commission set up to investigate doping in the IAAF, presided over by Richard Pound, founding President of WADA. This problem is by no means unique to sports drug control, having been identified as a significant issue for sports governance more broadly (Sherry & Shilbury, 2009; Sherry, Shilbury, & Wood, 2007).

Another example of where concerns about independence and conflict of interest emerge is the Court of Arbitration for Sport. Following observation over its relationship with the IOC, the International Council for the Arbitration for Sport was formed to take over the running of the Court of Arbitration for Sport. Of the 20 positions on the Board, 12 are chosen by Olympic organisations (e.g. the IOC, National Olympic Committees and Summer and Winter Olympic Federations), with the remaining eight chosen by the 12 members appointed by Olympic organisations. This creates two specific problems for claims of independence. The first is that Board members are appointed on the basis of a relationship with some aspect of Olympic administration. While the Swiss Federal Court has declared the Council and its Court to be independent relative to Swiss laws

(Reilly, 2012), it would be naive to think that this relationship would have no impact on the activity of the Council. The second is that for a Council whose use by non-Olympic sports is compelled by the Code (negating arguments that non-Olympic sports are at liberty to set up their own arbitration system), there is an absence of Board positions for those without a vested interest in the Olympic movement. As a result, the interests of non-Olympic sport are potentially compromised in relation to arbitration governance.

Representation

The governance of WADA includes taking advice from a range of committees. For example, the Athlete Committee provides advice to the Foundation Board on matters relating to athlete experiences of anti-doping. This seems a reasonable response to systemic governance democratisation concerns. However, like Board appointments, athletes are appointed undemocratically, and fail to account for any version of sport other than the elite level; for example, the views of non-elite sport are excluded (Donnelly, 2015). The failure of organisational governance in terms of representation is driven by the systemic governance mechanisms argued above. The implications of this failure and its impact on integrity for sport are demonstrated in professional cycling, where the precarious nature of employment and lack of employee protections for working conditions makes cyclists vulnerable to drug-based exploitation (Aubel & Ohl, 2014). The outcome for professional cyclists shows why robust athlete representation is needed in both sports drug control (e.g. how the relationship between athlete employees and sports employers can drive drug consumption) and sports governance generally (Kreft, 2011).

The concerns about representation magnify when considering claims athletes are chosen for their capacity to promote anti-doping rather than representing the views of all athletes (e.g. Schwab, 2014). The effect is that athlete voices opposing anti-doping or reflecting the experience of drug control outside elite professionalised sport are lost to both systemic and organisational governance. If this approach extends to other committees, it suggests manipulation of organisational governance that ultimately diminishes the integrity of drug control for sport (cf. Møller, 2014).

Boards and drug control

As noted above, it can be difficult to find audits or reviews of organisational governance processes in sport (Donnelly, 2015), and even more difficult to find audits or reviews of governance processes for drug control in sport. Australian sport has provided two reviews of organisational governance. The first arose following the admission of doping by several prominent Australian professional cyclists that prompted a review of governance in Cycling Australia (Woods, 2013). The second was a governance review in the early stages of the Essendon Supplements Saga (Switkowski, 2013). These rare reviews provide valuable insights into how boards respond to drug control issues within their sport. A third review emerged late in the course of writing this book, examining governance failures in relation to anti-doping in the IAAF.

Cycling Australia

The terms of reference for the Cycling Australia Review (CAR) (Woods, 2013) sought to understand the governance and administrative processes of the organisation, with attention given to its anti-doping policy and practices. What becomes apparent from the CAR is that the Board approached anti-doping as a compliance activity. That is, compliance with the Code was seen as sufficient to meet the obligations of the Code, enabling access to events and government funding. As a compliance cost, it is economically rational to minimise expenditure on drug control to deploy resources towards profit-making activities such as athletes and events (Sharpe, 2009). This was expressed by the Board's decision to respond to cycling's well-known drug control problems with a part-time manager to oversee the anti-doping activity of an organisation with 40,000 members. The Board was also criticised for relying on generic anti-doping education supplied by the Australian Sports Anti-Doping Authority (ASADA) rather than investing in cycling specific education for athletes or support personnel. The review concluded that Cycling Australia needed to re-categorise anti-doping as an essential cost of doing business that requires ongoing action among both line managers and the Board, rather than a rationally minimised compliance cost. It remains to be seen whether the recommendations of the review are to be audited.

Essendon Football Club

This case arose from claims by the Australian Crime Commission (2013) that organised crime was a critical threat to the Australian sports sector, and in particular the role of organised crime in doping. The report led to intense scrutiny of two professional sports clubs, the Essendon Football Club (Australian Football League) and the Cronulla Sharks (National Rugby League). In response to the claims, the Essendon Football Club undertook a voluntary review of governance (Switkowski, 2013). A number of key governance failures that saw the Board lose control of football operations were identified.

The problems were a consequence of failure to engage in appropriate oversight of football operations by the Board that saw a breakdown in leadership, transparency and accountability. Leadership was compromised in football operations with the introduction of a new coaching group that quickly strayed from 'business as usual' as personalities determined influence rather than position. For example, the marginalisation of medical staff and endorsement of sports science was seen as a particularly problematic breach of governance with regards to drug control. This created conflict within the organisation, and an unwillingness to communicate 'bad news' to the Board. This led to a decline in transparency and accountability across procurement of both goods (e.g. substances) and services (e.g. recruiting consultants), including a failure to engage in regular review and audit of football operation activities. As noted in the review, these issues could be resolved through minor changes in governance processes, such as including an agenda item that compels regular reporting and enables the Board to query football operations activity on a regular basis.

Outcomes of the Australian reviews

The two reviews lead to a conclusion that diminishes any enthusiasm that might arise from the successes arising from systemic governance; organisational governance of drug control for sport is seen as a compliance cost rather than a legitimate business activity. Further, Board members see the role of drugs in sport as one of many activities involved in running sports operations, and one that merits relatively little attention. This seems to be consistent with the evidence that drugs in sport issues have been managed in reaction to crises for much of its history (Ritchie, 2013). One explanation for this may be found in the literature around how well athletes and support personnel understand drug control for sport. Noting that many Board members are former athletes or support personnel, Board members probably have little understanding of the Code, assume they can handle it if it happens (Mazanov, Hemphill, Connor, Quirk, & Backhouse, 2015), and underestimate the need for drug control in their own sport while overestimating the need for other sports (Overbye & Wagner, 2014).

What becomes more concerning is the observation that these were two peak sports organisations in one of the most robust anti-doping nations in the world. The evidence indicates that, while policy harmonisation has worked for systemic governance, variation remains a feature of organisational governance (Hanstad, Skille, & Loland, 2010; Overbye & Wagner, 2013). The compliance based cost minimisation approach taken by well-resourced organisations brings into sharp focus whether sports organisations with fewer resources (e.g. semi-professional, non-elite or participation sport) have the capacity to develop effective governance of sports drug control (Henning & Dimeo, 2015). It is perhaps concerning that those working at the level of systemic governance are yet to address whether the systems designed to administer drug control are feasible beyond the rarefied world of elite professional sport (see Chapter 11). So while systemic governance has achieved breadth of compliance, it seems failures to address issues of organisational governance may explain the failure to achieve depth of compliance (Houlihan, 2014).

Independent Commission[1]

The Independent Commission (Pound, McLaren, & Younger, 2015) was formed in response to investigative journalists revealing systematic doping in Russian athletics. In terms of organisational governance, corruption appeared commonplace in the daily practice of anti-doping, from bribery (e.g. paying off doping control officers) to maladministration (e.g. lengthy delays and inconsistencies in administrative decisions). The Report suggested that both practices emerged due to a relatively indifferent attitude towards anti-doping governance. The corruption of governance mechanisms was also found at the highest levels of the IAAF, and was instrumental in sparking a change of leadership in that organisation, amid concerns to 'clean up' athletics.

The recommendations to resolve organisational governance focused on sanctioning those involved in corrupt practices and continuing to offer anti-doping education in Russia. The systemic governance recommendations were more sophisticated, aimed at attempting to get institutions to comply with the Code through the creation of more official positions (e.g. Chief Compliance Officer and Ombudsperson) and increases in reporting (e.g. to UNESCO). These have been designed to reinforce the role of WADA as a hegemonic regulator rather than a service provider.

Five key governance implications arise from the Independent Commission report. The first is that, like the Australian examples, anti-doping was accorded relatively low priority next to other performance outcomes, even at the highest levels of athletics. As a consequence, effort was directed at systemic compliance (achieving Code compliance) without regard for organisational compliance (preventing doping). The second is that, drawing on the Commission's expectation, the Russian athletics example is by no means isolated and the variation in organisational governance is likely to remain a feature of anti-doping. The third is that the recommendations suggest increasing the volume of governance mechanisms rather than looking to address whether the governance mechanisms in place are appropriate for the intended outcomes. The fourth implication was the fundamental failure in systemic governance monitoring practices to detect corruption. Finally, anti-doping governance is difficult even for the rarefied world of elite professional sport, which informs the prospects for success at other levels of sport.

The good and bad of governance for drugs in sport

The governance of drug control for sport has both positive and negative aspects. On the positive side, systemic governance has created a coherent network that facilitates institutional interaction around matters of drug control despite inheriting flaws from sports governance more generally. Unfortunately, these efforts have been let down by a failure to engage meaningfully with organisational governance. The democratisation flaw and problems with organisational governance suggest a critical threat to the attempt to use drug control to manage the integrity of sport. That is, governance failures in relation to drug control represent a risk to the trust relationship necessary to support the sports industry business model, especially efforts directed at leveraging CSR in sport (cf. Babiak & Wolfe, 2013). This bodes poorly for sports governance more broadly. The failure to integrate best-practice systemic and organisational governance indicates that sport still has a long way to go before being able to shed its unenviable reputation for poor governance.

That being said, the effect of policy harmonisation on systemic governance has created a system that could be adapted to deliver different models of drug control. This is particularly important given that the drug control system described only deals with doping. For example, a reinvention of drug control for sport may see WADA transformed into a World Sports Drug Agency (Mazanov, 2013) that responds to the sports drug matrix in full rather than in part (see Chapter 2). Such a change would require amendment rather than replacement of the existing approach, which could also address some of the other governance issues identified here (see Chapter 12). From this point of view, while the governance of drugs in sport is both good and bad, it provides a robust governance architecture that could serve as a platform for second generation sports drug control (Mazanov & Connor, 2010).

The general outcome is that integrity management cuts both ways. While integrity management may be seen as something that promotes trust, it also creates threats to trust. The governance failures of anti-doping (especially with regards to international athletics) threaten the trust producers and consumers have in both the production process and the mechanisms put in place to protect integrity. Thus, any attempt at integrity management in sport or other sectors needs to address the governance conundrum of 'who guards the guardians' (Møller, 2014). The danger lies in attempting to fix every administrative problem with a new set of governance mechanisms (e.g. Chief Compliance Officer and increased reporting obligations), inflating the costs of administration without having any effect on integrity (cf. Sharpe, 2009).

Note

1 As noted in the Addendum to Chapter 3, the Independent Commission could have been used as the focal case study for this book. Unfortunately, it was released when the writing of this book was in its final stages. It has been included here to acknowledge its importance as a significant event that informs drug control-led integrity management, and deserves far deeper analysis than was possible at the time of writing.

References

Australian Crime Commission (2013). *Organised Crime and Drugs in Sport*. Canberra: Commonwealth of Australia.

Althaus, C., Bridgman, P., & Davis, G. (2013). *The Australian Policy Handbook* (5th Ed.). Sydney: Allen & Unwin.

Aubel, O., & Ohl, F. (2014). An alternative approach to the prevention of doping in cycling. *International Journal of Drug Policy*, 25(6), 1094–1102.

Babiak, K., & Wolfe, R. (2013). Perspectives on corporate social responsibility in sport. In J. L. P. Paramio-Salcines, K. Babiak, & G. Walter (Eds.), *Routledge Handbook of Sport and Corporate Social Responsibility* (pp. 17–34). Abingdon: Routledge.

Bennett, D. (2013). Harm reduction and NFL drug policy. *Journal of Sport and Social Issues*, 37(2), 160–175.

Catlin, D. H., Fitch, K. D., & Ljungqvist, A. (2008). Medicine and science in the fight against doping in sport. *Journal of Internal Medicine*, 264(2), 99–114.

Camporesi, S., & Knuckles, J. A. (2014). Shifting the burden of proof in doping: Lessons from environmental sustainability applied to high-performance sport. *Reflective Practice*, 15(1), 106–118.

Camporesi, S., & McNamee, M. J. (2014). Performance enhancement, elite athletes and anti-doping governance: Comparing human guinea pigs in pharmaceutical research and professional sports. *Philosophy, Ethics, and Humanities in Medicine*, 9(1), 4.

Donnelly, P. (2015). What if the players controlled the game? Dealing with the consequences of the crisis of governance in sports. *European Journal for Sport and Society*, 12(1), 11–30.

Ferkins, L., & Shilbury, D. (2012). Good boards are strategic: What does that mean for sport governance? *Journal of Sport Management*, 26(1), 67–80.

Ferkins, L., & Shilbury, D. (2015). Board strategic balance: An emerging sport governance theory. *Sport Management Review*, 18(4), 489–500.

Ferkins, D., & van Bottenburg, M. (2013). The governance of high performance sport. In P. Sotiriadou, & V. De Bosscher (Eds.), *Managing High Performance Sport* (pp. 115–136). Abingdon: Routledge.

Geeraert, A., Alm, J., & Groll, M. (2014). Good governance in international sport organizations: An analysis of the 35 Olympic sport governing bodies. *International Journal of Sport Policy and Politics*, 6(3), 281–306.

Hanstad, D. V., Skille, E. Å., & Loland, S. (2010). Harmonization of anti-doping work: Myth or reality? *Sport in Society*, 13(3), 418–430.

Henne, K. (2015). *Testing for Athlete Citizenship*. Rutgers University Press: New Brunswick, NJ.

Henning, A. D., & Dimeo, P. (2015). Questions of fairness and anti-doping in US cycling: The contrasting experiences of professionals and amateurs. *Drugs: Education, Prevention and Policy*, 22(5), 400–409.

Houlihan, B. (2004). Civil rights, doping control and the world anti-doping code. *Sport in Society*, 7(3), 420–437.

Houlihan, B. (2014). Achieving compliance in international anti-doping policy: An analysis of the 2009 World Anti-Doping Code. *Sport Management Review*, 17(3), 265–276.

Jedlicka, S. (2014). The normative discourse of anti-doping policy. *International Journal of Sport Policy and Politics*, 6(3), 429–442.

Kornbeck, J. (2013). The naked spirit of sport: a framework for revisiting the system of bans and justifications in the world anti-doping code. *Sport, Ethics and Philosophy*, 7(3), 313–330.

Kreft, L. (2011). Elite sportspersons and commodity control: anti-doping as quality assurance. *International Journal of Sport Policy and Politics*, 3(2), 151–161.

Kustec Lipicer, S., & McArdle, D. (2014). National law, domestic governance and global policy: A case study of anti-doping policy in Slovenia. *International Journal of Sport Policy and Politics*, 6(1), 71–87.

MacAloon, J. J. (2011). Scandal and governance: inside and outside the IOC 2000 Commission. *Sport in Society*, 14(3), 292–308.

MacGregor, O., Griffith, R., Ruggiu, D., & McNamee, M. (2013). Anti-doping, purported rights to privacy and WADA's whereabouts requirements: A legal analysis. *Fair Play*, 1(2), 13–38.

Magdalinksi, T. (2009). *Sport, Technology and the Body*. Abingdon: Routledge.

Malloy, D. C., & Zakus, D. H. (2002). Ethics of drug testing in sport – an invasion of privacy justified? *Sport, Education and Society*, 7(2), 203–218.

Mazanov, J. (2013). *Vale WADA, ave 'World Sports Drug Agency'*. Performance Enhancement & Health, 2(2), 80–83.

Mazanov, J. (2014). Drug control in sport: Who and how. In B. Stewart, & M. Burke (Eds.), *Drugs and Sport: Writings from the Edge* (pp. 33–71). Melbourne, Australia: Dry Ink Press.

Mazanov, J., & Connor, J. (2010). Rethinking the management of drugs in sport. *International Journal of Sport Policy*, 2(1), 49–63.

Mazanov, J., Hemphill, D., Connor, J., Quirk, F., & Backhouse, S. H. (2015). Australian athlete support personnel lived experience of anti-doping. *Sport Management Review*, 18(2), 218–230.

McNamee, M. J., & Fleming, S. (2007). Ethics audits and corporate governance: The case of public sector sports organizations. *Journal of Business Ethics*, 73(4), 425–437.

Miller, S. (2011). Good governance and anti-doping policy: An international federation view. *International Journal of Sport Policy and Politics*, 3(2), 279–288.

Mitten, M. J., & Opie, H. (2010). Sports law: Implications for the development of international, comparative, and national law and global dispute resolution. *Tulane Law Review*, 85(2), 269–322.

Møller, V. (2014). Who guards the guardians? *International Journal of the History of Sport*, 31(8), 934–950.

Overbye, M. (2016). Doping control in sport: An investigation of how elite athletes perceive and trust the functioning of the doping testing system in their sport. *Sport Management Review, 19*(1), 6–22.

Overbye, M., & Wagner, U. (2013). Between medical treatment and performance enhancement: An investigation of how elite athletes experience Therapeutic Use Exemptions. *International Journal of Drug Policy, 24*(6), 579–588.

Overbye, M., & Wagner, U. (2014). Experiences, attitudes and trust: An inquiry into elite athletes' perception of the whereabouts reporting system. *International Journal of Sport Policy and Politics, 6*(3), 407–428.

Park, J. K. (2005). Governing doped bodies: The world anti-doping agency and the global culture of surveillance. *Cultural Studies Critical Methodologies, 5*(2), 174–188.

Parks, J. (2013). 'Nothing but trouble': The Soviet Union's push to 'Democratise' international sports during the Cold War, 1959–1962. *The International Journal of the History of Sport, 30*(13), 1554–1567.

Pound, R., McLaren, R., & Younger, G. (2015). *Independent Commission Report #1*. Montreal: World Anti-Doping Agency.

Rabin, O. (2011). Involvement of the health industry in the fight against doping in sport. *Forensic Science International, 213*(1), 10–14.

Reilly, L. (2012). An introduction to the Court of Arbitration for Sport (CAS) and the role of National Courts in international sports disputes. *Journal of Dispute Resolution, 2012*(1), 63–81.

Ritchie, I. (2013). The construction of a policy: The World Anti-Doping Code's 'spirit of sport' clause. *Performance Enhancement and Health, 2*(4), 194–200.

Rowbottom, M. (2013). *Foul Play: The Dark Arts of Cheating in Sport*. London: Bloomsbury.

Schwab, B. (2014). Why Australian sport must cut its ties with WADA. Sydney Morning Herald, 15 June 2014. Available at: www.smh.com.au/sport/why-australian-sports-must-cut-ties-with-wada-20140615-zs8k1.html (accessed 7 August 2015).

Sharpe, K. (2009). The economics of drugs in sport. *Sport in Society, 12*(3), 344–355.

Sherry, E., & Shilbury, D. (2009). Board directors and conflict of interest: A study of a sport league. *European Sport Management Quarterly, 9*(1), 47–62.

Sherry, E., Shilbury, D., & Wood, G. (2007). Wrestling with 'conflict of interest' in sport management. *Corporate Governance, 7*(3), 267–277.

Sottas, P. E., & Vernec, A. (2012). Current implementation and future of the Athlete Biological Passport. *Bioanalysis, 4*(13), 1645–1652.

Switkowski, Z. (2013). *Review of Essendon Football Club Governance*. Available at: www.essendonfc.com.au/news/2013-05-06/dr-ziggy-switkowski-report (accessed 23 February 2016).

Waddington, I. (2010). Surveillance and control in sport: A sociologist looks at the WADA whereabouts system. *International Journal of Sport Policy, 2*(3), 255–274.

Warren, I., Palmer, D., & Whelan, C. (2014). Surveillance, governance and professional sport. *Surveillance and Society, 11*(4), 439–453.

Woods, J. (2013). *Review of Cycling Australia – Final Report*. Canberra: Commonwealth of Australia.

Chapter 8

Managing drug risks in sport

The integration of drugs with modern sport compels the management of risks arising from that integration. Risk management of drugs in sport can be broadly divided into two categories. The first is the attempt to manage the relationship sport has with drugs in terms of the classification system offered in Chapter 2. The second is the need to manage the risks introduced by the anti-doping policy. Anti-doping forces sports managers to strategise both the role of drugs and anti-doping compliance in their programmes. Anti-doping also introduces resourcing dilemmas for sports programme operations (e.g. investing in anti-doping education).

How risk and risk management are understood has changed considerably over time. The meaning of risk changed from 'chance to danger' as part of a general cultural evolution in the understanding of the term. This transition emerged from early work mathematising gambling probabilities in the seventeenth century, to marine insurance in the eighteenth century to an economic understanding of risk in the nineteenth century (Douglas, 1990). The rational understanding of risk and risk management has since become entrenched in science and manufacturing (Douglas, 1990, p. 2), leading to a proliferation of socially and politically motivated definitions, research and tools (Beck, 1992) designed to inform management of risk across market sectors. Within sport, risk management has been applied to managing sports-related health risks (e.g. Fuller & Drawer, 2004; Fuller, Junge, & Dvorak, 2012), operational risk management (Appenzeller, 2012) and event risk management (e.g. Hanstad, 2012; Leopkey & Parent, 2009).

Drug risks

Following the typology offered in Chapter 2, the risks associated with each class of drug are evaluated in terms of their implications for integrity management in sport. The risks outlined are by no means a comprehensive examination by class of drug. Instead, they present risks that serve as a starting point to inform future examination of the risks arising from the interaction between sport and drugs. Chapter 11 expands this discussion by examining the apparent lack of meaningful drug risk management in non-elite, non-male sport.

For the purposes of the current discussion, over-the-counter and prescription drugs have been combined on the grounds that they are typically manufactured by the same pharmaceutical companies. Doping is treated is a separate case.

Licit drugs

Sport's relationship with licit drugs, outlined in Chapters 2 and 3, provides a template for understanding the relationship with other drugs, and in particular tobacco and alcohol. The history of sport's relationship with tobacco and alcohol demonstrates how violation of rules- and values-based expectations can be significant risks for sport. This history shows that failure to adequately manage the relationship with drug companies sees sport risk external regulation, with all the costs that implies (see Chapter 5 and below). For example, the outcome of the relationship with tobacco indicates sport needs to be mindful of its role in health promotion and expectations around advertising and children (see Chapters 3 and 10). Learning from the experience with tobacco, sport needs to amend its relationship with alcohol to promote use rather than misuse or abuse (values-based) and voluntarily limit the nature of alcohol sponsorship to avoid exposing children to alcohol-related advertising (rules-based). It remains to be seen whether sport has matured enough following its relationship with tobacco to engage in such drug control-led risk management of integrity with alcohol (cf. Crompton, 2014; Hanstad & Waddington, 2009).

Sports-related misuse and abuse of alcohol remains, in the author's opinion, the most significant drug risk to sport. In simple terms, athletes consume alcohol in more dangerous ways than the general population (Green, Nelson, & Hartmann, 2014; Kwan, Bobko, Faulkner, Donnelly, & Cairney, 2014). Further, the correlation between sports consumption (e.g. attending events or watching broadcasts) and alcohol misuse and abuse remains a significant risk for sport (e.g. Dearing et al., 2014; Palmer, 2011). The misuse and abuse of alcohol creates risk across the sports industry, from athlete and fan health and well-being (violence, vandalism and rape), to sports managers handling alcohol-fuelled scandals, to government public health interventions. As argued in Chapter 1, given the close association between sport and dangerous drinking, sport has an obligation to the societies it inhabits to address its relationship with alcohol (see also Lyne & Galloway, 2012). However, given alcohol occupies such a central role in sport, the risk needs to be managed rather than eliminated. For example, there is evidence that aggressive approaches to alcohol control in sport (e.g. zero tolerance) have a negative impact on attendance and revenues (e.g. Mentha & Wakerman, 2009). As a result, sport needs to mitigate the risks associated with the culture of alcohol misuse and abuse in sport by building a culture of alcohol use (see Chapters 2 and 3).

Supplements

The primary integrity risk to sport arising from its relationship with the supplements industry stems from potential violations of producer and consumer expectations undermining trust in the sports sector. The first potential violation comes from the unsubstantiated claims made by many supplements (see Chapter 5). The danger to sport emerges when athlete or sports programme endorsement (either through consumption or sponsorship) is seen to legitimise claims about a supplement. The risk is realised when the supplement has no or undesirable effects, potentially undermining the trust relationship.

Inaccurate labelling of supplements (e.g. active ingredients only, ingredients of interest to advertised claims, or incorrect ingredients) represents a potential risk to sport that needs to be managed. The risks associated with inaccurate labelling are that it makes it difficult for sports producers or consumers to know what they are ingesting (e.g. Petróczi, Taylor, & Naughton, 2011; Pomeranz, Munsell, & Harris, 2013). For some products, mislabelling may be intentional to promote sales or a result of poor quality controls during manufacturing. The latter point may lead to the absence of active ingredients (meaning the supplement has no effect, or potentially the wrong effect) or the contamination of supplements with prescription or illicit drugs (see Chapter 2). The consequences of this risk become more apparent when considering an adolescent who consumes large amounts of supplements contaminated by a combination of anabolic steroids and methamphetamines. As a result, sport needs to take an interest in the risks associated with both supplement labelling and manufacturing.

Beyond supplement production, the speed with which the supplements market evolves represents a risk to producers and consumers. The increasing number of entrants to an already cluttered market can make it difficult for producers and consumers to determine which products reliably meet their needs. This creates a risk for producers looking for supplements to influence sports performance having to pay for specialist advice (cost), learn about supplements (time), consume the supplements without being informed (no effect or contaminated), or abstain and lose potential benefits (recovery or performance).

One obvious answer is regulation; for example, the Australian Senate (2013) has considered submissions arguing for the regulation of the term 'sports supplement' to give assurance of evidence for claims, labelling and manufacturing standards. The supplements industry has so far successfully resisted calls for government regulation (Starr, 2015). However, there is evidence to suggest that marketised regulation has begun to emerge with an increasing number of organisations specialising in third party quality assurance certification for supplements (e.g. NSF and Informed Sport). It remains to be seen whether such third party regulation leads to improvements in claims, labelling and manufacturing to mitigate the risks to sport, or whether the integrity of the supplement certification industry can itself be trusted (e.g. certification based on commercial relationships rather than supplement quality).

While the third party regulation experiment runs its course, it may be valuable for sport to still consider establishing model policies for engaging with supplements manufacturers around the integrity concerns outlined. This would be an astute move given governments have already indicated their willingness to adopt model policy from sport in relation to drug control (e.g. anti-doping).

Over-the-counter and prescription drugs

Given the average elite athlete competes with 2.5–3.0 drugs in their system (see Chapter 1) sport needs to manage the risks arising from the pharmaceutical industry. Government regulation of the pharmaceutical industry provides a framework for managing some risks. However, there are still some risks that managers need to be explicitly aware of. These include the pharmaceutical industry taking advantage of sports programme and athlete willingness to trial new drugs yet to appear on the Prohibited List, and how the pharmaceutical industry might manipulate a drug appearing on the Prohibited List for commercial reasons.

There is potential for exploitation of athletes as 'guinea pigs' in pharmaceutical trials. King and Robeson (2007) observe that both athletes and sports programmes take great interest in drug-based innovation; where athletes and sports programmes feel they can derive some competitive advantage (e.g. injury prevention, improved recovery or performance) they will offer to trial the drug, potentially more so when that drug is absent from the Prohibited List. King and Robeson note that drug trialling in sports settings appears to overlook the well-established standards and protections of clinical trial protocols. They also observe there is a risk that the sports programme acts in the interests of the programme rather than the interests of the individual athlete (promoting institutional interests at the expense of individual interest; see Chapter 7), and coerces athletes into taking drugs they would otherwise abstain from. Camporesi and McNamee (2014) expand on the potential risks by pointing out the significant risks that such trialling poses to athletes, including the breadth of 'chemical cocktails' athlete bodies are exposed to over their careers. The interactions of these different drugs and the effects of those interactions on athlete health represent risks that need to be addressed. As a consequence, sport needs to ensure that any drug trials are conducted in a rigorous manner that protects the integrity of the athlete, both in terms of individual trials and the number of trials an athlete might participate in over the course of their career.

The moral panic around the role of drugs in sport (Crichter, 2014; McDermott, 2016) means that sport has to be very careful about how it manages its relationship with the pharmaceutical industry. A troubling risk emerges from the management of the Prohibited List. As argued elsewhere (Chapters 4, 6 and 7), there is a level of uncertainty as to the basis upon which a drug appears on the Prohibited List, both in terms of the definition and lack of transparency in decision making. Drug companies would be understandably very interested in whether one of their products might appear on the Prohibited List with an eye to the impact on sales either negatively (e.g. the drug becomes seen as immoral) or positively (e.g. increasing sales through the expanding black market; Fincouer, van de Ven, & Mulrooney, 2015; Paoli & Donati, 2014). For example, sales of meldonium in Russia doubled in the weeks after tennis star Maria Sharapova admitted its use during a crackdown on the use of the drug by the World Anti-Doping Agency in early 2016 (ABC, 2016). Doubling sales volume means pharmaceutical companies may take a great interest in manipulating whether their or a competitor's drug appears on the Prohibited List. Given the demonstrated level of corruption in sports governance where decision making lacks transparency (e.g. IOC and FIFA bid scandals, and doping in the UCI and IAAF) and questionable drug approval practices in the pharmaceutical industry (Braithwaite, 2013; Flaherty, 2013), the lack of transparency increases the risk of corruption in prohibition decisions to protect a drug from listing, listing a drug to improve sales, or disrupting a competitor's drug through listing (industrial sabotage). Corruption of a process designed to protect the integrity of sport represents a significant risk (see Chapter 7).

These two examples demonstrate that sport needs to establish rigorous governance mechanisms to mitigate risks stemming from engagement with the pharmaceutical industry. This has been recognised, to some extent, in response to interactions between the industries to promote the anti-doping ideology (e.g. Elliott & Leishman, 2012; Rabin, 2011). As argued in Chapter 7, the developing administrative lingua franca emerging from systemic governance of anti-doping may provide a basis upon which to mitigate risks arising from interactions between the sport and pharmaceutical industries of the kind raised here. For example, a stronger relationship may see more rigorous administration of drug trials in sporting contexts and greater interest in transparent prohibition of drugs.

Illicit drugs

Three potential risks to the integrity of sport arising from illicit drugs are addressed. The first looks to the management of athletes who consume illicit drugs. The second covers the integrity risks associated with prohibiting illicit drugs under the World Anti-Doping Code (the Code). The third risk relates to risk management of illicit drug testing programmes in non-elite sport.

As noted in Chapter 3, the genesis of drug control in United States professional sport emerged, in part, in response to athlete consumption of illicit drugs. It is also well understood that some athletes end up misusing or abusing illicit drugs irrespective of prevention activity. Athletes who are also illicit drug addicts create a difficult contradiction between the great sporting myth (athletes as custodians and guardians of what makes sport 'good') and cultural constructions of drug addicts (morally deviant and compulsive victims) (Seear & Frazer, 2010) that threatens the integrity of sport. This risk is mitigated following health-based harm-minimisation principles (see Chapter 4) by reinterpreting the addicted athlete as a 'fallen hero' with an illness that needs treatment. In elite sport, there are usually limited opportunities for an athlete to receive drug treatment managed by their sport before their contract is terminated (e.g. the Australian Football League's three strike policy; Stewart, Adair, & Smith, 2011). If the athlete fails to overcome their drug addiction, the integrity of sport is preserved for having followed both the rules (employment contract) and values (supporting the athlete), and the relationship between sport and the athlete can be concluded. In non-elite sport, scarcity of funding means risks associated with athlete illicit drug addiction are transferred to other sectors for treatment (e.g. public drug treatment programmes). This demonstrates that sport has a well-established approach to managing the integrity risks associated with illicit drug addiction among athletes; whether that approach is ethical or effective is beyond the scope of this chapter.

The second risk emerges from violations of expectations associated with managing illicit drugs that are governed by the Code. While illicit drugs policies tend to follow harm-minimisation principles, the introduction of anti-doping has complicated whether those principles can be followed. By appearing on the in-competition Prohibited List, an athlete addicted to cocaine (prohibited as a stimulant) is subject to the Code. While sanctioning an athlete under the Code is consistent with rules-based integrity, there is a risk that this is inconsistent with values-based expectations (e.g. natural justice expectations to support the 'fallen hero') (cf. Smith, Stavros, Westberg, Wilson, & Boyle, 2013). The evidence indicates that sports producers have strong values-based expectations about drug control in sport which departs from the rules, including a preference for harm-minimisation principles in relation to illicit drug control in sport and challenging the prohibition of illicit drugs under the Code (Mazanov, Hemphill, Connor, Quirk, & Backhouse, 2015). This divergence in expectations about how sport should address illicit drug management has sparked debate over whether illicit drugs should appear on the Prohibited List (Henne, Koh, & McDermott, 2013; Waddington, Christiansen, Gleaves, Hoberman, & Møller, 2013). The divergence between the preference for harm-minimisation in relation to illicit drugs and punitive prohibition for doping represents a potential risk to the integrity of sport, making managing the risk a difficult task of reconciling different ideological approaches to managing drugs in sport.

Where elite sport tends towards having sophisticated drug testing protocols that have emerged from legal challenges to anti-doping protocols, non-elite sports' interest in testing for illicit drugs (for a variety of reasons) is less well developed. For example, Spengler, Connaughton, and Pittman (2006) go into some detail on how to mitigate the legal risks associated with illicit drug testing in recreational or school sports in the United States. Appenzeller (2012) follows a similar strategy in addressing illicit drug testing in the National Collegiate Athletic Association. In defending against legal risks, they emphasise rigorous policy (including Codes of Conduct; although see Chapter 9 for more on this point), clear procedures, a strong information campaign and taking care with regards to coercion (e.g. participation is dependent upon submitting to an illicit drug test). Illicit drug testing outside elite sport begins to take on the character of workplace drug testing, with all the risk management that implies (e.g. Verstraete, 2011).

Managing risks from doping and anti-doping

The risks associated with doping and anti-doping in sport are assessed from two points of view. The first is through game-theoretic accounts of doping. The second draws on resourcing dilemmas. Further discussion of risks raised in this section occurs in Chapters 9 and 11.

The doping game

Drug consumption to influence sports performance creates a set of strategic games for both athletes and managers. The introduction of anti-doping complicates the strategic game. While doping-games have been examined from the athlete's point of view, the results from athlete games can be extrapolated to explore how managers may strategise drug use across sports programmes.

The most basic doping game refers to use of a performance enhancing drug in a symmetric (both players adopt the same strategy) two-person contest characterised by the Prisoner's Dilemma (Berensten, 2002; Breivik, 1987). Core assumptions at this point are that the athlete wants to win the competition (Lombardian) and thinks doping will influence the outcome of the competition. The athlete has to decide whether to dope without knowing whether their competitor has doped. If neither or both dope the outcome of the competition is uncertain, but if one dopes the outcome is certain. The outcome of the game across strategies (e.g. Lombardian, Machiavellian or Brownian) is doping (Breivik, 1987). The outcome changes slightly by increasing the number of athletes and strategies (where athletes play asymmetric games), although doping still appears to be a dominant strategy (Breivik, 1992; Eber, 2008).

The introduction of anti-doping complicates the game as athletes need to introduce the likelihood of their doping being detected. While the evidence suggests that the likelihood of accurate drug test-based detection is surprisingly low (Berry, 2008; Pitsch, 2009), the introduction of analytic (drug test) and non-analytic (e.g. circumstantial evidence) detection methods means athletes still have to consider the likelihood of detection. Even with detection taken into account, the Nash equilibrium is still for athletes to dope (Haugen, 2004). From a risk management perspective, inducing a doping-free equilibrium only occurs with the introduction of alternative outcomes, such as health consequences, punishments or prize money (Haugen, Nepusz, & Petróczi, 2013; Kräkel, 2007). However, the role of punishment is likely to have a limited effect on athlete behaviour (Kirstein, 2014), and would only likely work for a severe prohibitionist model of the kind proposed in Chapter 3 (see Hirschmann, 2015). As a result, managers need to make decisions about how to manage athlete doping relative to pay offs such as health or prize money. The recommendations arising from athlete doping-games typically refer to increasing the likelihood of detection (e.g. whistle-blowing) and changing the ratio of financial penalties (either increasing fines or decreasing prize money) to induce doping-free sport. While such theoretical analyses make valuable contributions, it is yet to be established whether such suggestions are also practical across stakeholders. For example, the lag between the introduction of a new drug and the development of a reliable drug test (Mazanov & McDermott, 2009) means that increasing the likelihood of detection through drug testing is impractical.

Managers also have to play doping-games with sports programmes to access the benefits of doping and anti-doping (see Fincouer et al., 2015, for an example of this from elite cycling). Noting that game-theoretic analyses of how sports managers strategise doping within their programme are yet to be established, the following presents the basis for a starting set of assumptions that might guide such analysis.

The ideal situation for a manager is to have different groups of athletes under different doping regimes; one group that abstains from all drugs (no risk of sanction), one group that works within anti-doping (low risk), one group that works at the margins of anti-doping (medium risk), and one group that ignores anti-doping (high risk). This approach enables perform-ance managers to access the benefits of doping without the entire pro-gramme being eliminated from competition. This would work for well-funded swimming or athletics programmes, but may be more difficult for less well-funded programmes or team sports. Where managers have to adopt a single approach, the decision relates to how much risk they are willing to take with their programmes. The Essendon Football Club's experience with an 'experimental supplements programme' suggests that high-risk doping is cheaper to administer over the long term. Essendon's supplements programme was at the margins of anti-doping, with ambigu-ity whether the drugs in question qualified as doping. This brought with it a range of direct and indirect costs (see Chapter 5) that arose from, among other things, innovation costs and the costs of having to determine whether the innovation violated anti-doping. In hindsight, it would have been cheaper to avoid innovation and use drugs with known performance enhancing effects in clear violation of the policy. That way, if detected, the violation would have been resolved quickly rather than damaging the club across several seasons.

Programme managers also need to game anti-doping in terms of com-petitors. Like the athlete doping game, managers choose a drug strategy based on estimating the risk their or another programme is likely to be sanctioned for doping. For example, when planning a season, a manager may include the relative risk of a programme anticipated to place more highly in a competition being disqualified as a result of a medium or high-risk doping strategy (as happened to Essendon in the 2013 season). The manager then has to decide whether to compete in terms of adopting a similarly risky doping strategy (keeping in mind performance incentives in employment contracts; see Chapter 9), or adopting a low or no risk strategy on the basis that the other programme is disqualified. Asymmetries emerge when adding the 'cat-and-mouse' element to the game, where man-agers may seek to increase the chances of sanctions being imposed against a competitor through manipulating the media or anonymous tip-offs, and have to assume others are doing so to their programme (industrial espionage).

In addition to strategising the doping within and between programmes, managers also need to manage the risk associated with consumer responses to doping. Game-theoretic models of how consumers respond to doping indicate they are likely to turn away from sport if there is too much emphasis on making a public spectacle of athletes found to have doped (detection-based deterrence) (Buechel, Emrich, & Pohlkamp, 2014). This leads to the counterintuitive implication that sports managers need to catch enough athlete doping to convince consumers of drug control-led integrity management without catching too many and undermining consumer trust in sport production. There is evidence that this is exactly what happens, with the average 2 per cent sanction rate for anti-doping rule violations argued to optimise the economic value of sporting events for consumers, organisers and athletes (Frenger, Emrich, & Pitsch, 2013). One interpretation of this result is that the US$500 million annual price tag of anti-doping means sport can enjoy the benefits of drug control-led integrity management, and also enjoy the benefits of doping in sport (e.g. more attractive sporting spectacles such as breaking world records).

Resourcing doping and anti-doping

Irrespective of the strategy managers choose to employ, doping and anti-doping represent necessary costs to compete in sporting events (Sharpe, 2009). Anti-doping compliance is addressed first, as it is a cost that is borne by all sport to access events, from wealthy professional sports through to volunteer-only non-elite sport (see Chapter 11 for more on this point). As argued in Chapter 7, sports managers seek to minimise investment in anti-doping to achieve the compliance necessary to access events, such as trading off the cost of communicating doping policy updates against paying a premium for supplements certified as contaminant free (anti-doping compliant) that support athlete performance. The essential dilemma for managers is to work out the point of diminishing returns, as investment in anti-doping compliance past a certain point is unlikely to lead to better outcomes, especially with regards to issues like anti-doping education (see Chapter 9). The risk is that too little investment makes the programme vulnerable to doping-related sanctions, and that too much reduces the resources available to profit-making activities.

Resourcing doping refers to the management of drugs to enhance sports performance that are both legitimate (e.g. caffeine) and prohibited (e.g. anabolic steroids). In wealthy elite sports, the increasingly complex nature of drug-based performance enhancement in sport means managers have to secure the services of highly qualified personnel (e.g. sports nutritionists, sports physicians and sports scientists), which brings other risks (see Chapter 9). Further, the nature of doping production and supply (e.g. contaminated supplements) means that managers have to expend resources quality assuring the drugs they do bring into a sports programme (e.g. paying a premium to purchase certified products, or paying for quality assurance). By comparison, poorer elite sports and non-elite sport are often left to navigate such issues without specialist advice or support, increasing the risk of sanction (see Chapter 11). Like anti-doping, the risk of investing too little means potentially being uncompetitive with athletes or programmes that do invest more in managing doping (either in terms of performance or being sanctioned).

Managing the integrity risks of drugs in sport

The brief overview of integrity risks associated with managing drugs in sport indicates a surprising breadth of issues. Reflecting on the breadth of issues raises a concern about whether there is also a risk in emphasising management of doping at the expense of other drugs. For example, anti-doping may lead to an underestimation of the risk alcohol poses to the integrity of sport. Reflecting on anti-doping specifically, it creates new risks to the integrity of sport arising from policy contradictions (illicit drugs) through to creating incentives to engage in corrupt behaviour (e.g. drug prohibition or sabotaging competitors). As a result, while it is clearly appropriate to engage in drug control-led integrity management, it may be necessary to re-examine those risks to determine which can be eliminated (e.g. governance) and which represent the greatest threat to the integrity of sport.

The outcome for integrity management more generally is to anticipate how regulation changes the nature of risk. For example, the introduction of anti-doping changed the nature of how drugs are strategised rather than changing whether drugs were used. The game-theoretic accounts of doping indicate that the underlying nature of the game (e.g. incentives and deterrents) needs to be fundamentally changed to motivate the desired behaviour (cf. Fife-Schaw & Abraham, 2009). This suggests that a deeper consideration is needed of whether regulation that creates opportunities to game the system (attempting to control existing behaviour) or whether restructuring the game's parameters (creating new behaviours) is the best way to manage integrity. While the latter may lead to better control over integrity, the former is more realistic, especially when it comes to entrenched traditions of sport.

References

ABC (2016). Meldonium sales double in Russia after Maria Sharapova scandal, survey finds. Available at: www.abc.net.au/news/2016-03-19/russian-sales-of-meldonium-double:-survey/7260234 (accessed 25 March 2016).

Appenzeller, H. (Ed.). (2012). *Risk Management in Sport: Issues and Strategies (3rd Ed)*. Durham, NC: Carolina Academic Press.

Australian Senate (2013). *Practice of Sports Science in Australia* (Submission 1). Canberra: Commonwealth of Australia.

Beck, U. (1992). *Risk Society: Towards a New Modernity*. London: Sage Publications.

Berensten, A. (2002). The economics of doping. *European Journal of Political Economy*, 18(4), 109–127.

Berry, D. A. (2008). The science of doping. *Nature*, 454(7205), 692–693.

Buechel, B., Emrich, E., & Pohlkamp, S. (2014). Nobody's innocent: The role of customers in the doping dilemma. *Journal of Sports Economics*, 3(1), 90–96.

Braithwaite, J. (2013). *Corporate Crime in the Pharmaceutical Industry*. Oxon: Routledge.

Breivik, G. (1987). The doping dilemma. Some game theoretical and philosophical considerations. *Sportwissenschaft*, *17*(1), 83–94.

Breivik, G. (1992). Doping games a game theoretical exploration of doping. *International Review for the Sociology of Sport*, *27*(3), 235–253.

Camporesi, S., & McNamee, M. J. (2014). Performance enhancement, elite athletes and anti-doping governance: Comparing human guinea pigs in pharmaceutical research and professional sports. *Philosophy, Ethics, and Humanities in Medicine*, *9*(4).

Crichter, C. (2014). New perspectives on anti-doping policy: From moral panic to moral regulation. *International Journal of Sport Policy and Politics*, *6*(2), 153–169.

Crompton, J. L. (2014). Potential negative outcomes from sponsorship for a sport property. *Managing Leisure*, *19*(6), 420–441.

Dearing, R. L., Twaragowski, C. L., Smith, P. H., Homish, G. G., Connors, G. J., & Walitzer, K. S. (2014). Super Bowl Sunday: Risky business for at-risk (male) drinkers? *Substance Use and Misuse*, *49*(10), 1359–1363.

Douglas, M. (1990). Risk as a forensic resource. *Daedalus*, *119*(4), 1–16.

Eber, N. (2008). The performance-enhancing drug game reconsidered: A fair play approach. *Journal of Sports Economics*, *9*(3), 318–327.

Elliott, S., & Leishman, B. (2012). Abuse of medicines for performance enhancement in sport: Why is this a problem for the pharmaceutical industry? *Bioanalysis*, *4*(13), 1681–1690.

Fife-Schaw, C., & Abraham, C. (2009). How much behaviour change should we expect from health promotion campaigns targeting cognitions? An approach to pre-intervention assessment. *Psychology and Health*, *24*(7), 763–776.

Fincouer, B., van de Ven, K., & Mulrooney, K. (2015). The symbiotic evolution of anti-doping and supply chains of doping substances: How criminal networks may benefit from anti-doping policy. *Trends in Organized Crime*, *18*(3), 229–250.

Flaherty, D. K. (2013). Ghost-and guest-authored pharmaceutical industry-sponsored studies: Abuse of academic integrity, the peer review system, and public trust. *Annals of Pharmacotherapy*, *47*(7–8), 1081–1083.

Frenger, M., Emrich, E., & Pitsch, W. (2013). How to produce the belief in clean sports which sells. *Performance Enhancement and Health*, *2*(4), 210–215.

Fuller, C., & Drawer, S. (2004). The application of risk management in sport. *Sports Medicine*, *34*(6), 349–356.

Fuller, C. W., Junge, A., & Dvorak, J. (2012). Risk management: FIFA's approach for protecting the health of football players. *British Journal of Sports Medicine*, *46*(1), 11–17.

Green, K., Nelson, T. F., & Hartmann, D. (2014). Binge drinking and sports participation in college: Patterns among athletes and former athletes. *International Review for the Sociology of Sport*, *49*(3–4), 417–434.

Hanstad, D. V. (2012). Risk management in major sporting events: A participating national Olympic team's perspective. *Event Management*, *16*(3), 189–201.

Hanstad, D. V., & Waddington, I. (2009). Sport, health and drugs: A critical re-examination of some key issues and problems. *Perspectives in Public Health*, *129*(4), 174–182.

Haugen, K. K. (2004). The performance-enhancing drug game. *Journal of Sports Economics*, 5(1), 67–86.

Haugen, K. K., Nepusz, T., & Petróczi, A. (2013). The multi-player performance-enhancing drug game. *PLoS ONE*, 8(5), e63306.

Henne, K., Koh, B., & McDermott, V. (2013). Coherence of drug policy in sports: Illicit inclusions and illegal inconsistencies. *Performance Enhancement and Health*, 2(2), 48–55.

Hirschmann, D. (2015). May increasing doping sanctions discourage entry to the competition? *Journal of Sports Economics*. DOI: 1527002515595265

King, N. M., & Robeson, R. (2007). Athlete or guinea pig? Sports and enhancement research. *Studies in Ethics, Law, and Technology*, 1(1).

Kirstein, R. (2014). Doping, the inspection game, and Bayesian enforcement. *Journal of Sports Economics*, 15(4), 385–409.

Kräkel, M. (2007). Doping and cheating in contest-like situations. *European Journal of Political Economy*, 23(4), 988–1006.

Kwan, M., Bobko, S., Faulkner, G., Donnelly, P., & Cairney, J. (2014). Sport participation and alcohol and illicit drug use in adolescents and young adults: A systematic review of longitudinal studies. *Addictive Behaviors*, 39(3), 497–506.

Leopkey, B., & Parent, M. M. (2009). Risk management issues in large-scale sporting events: A stakeholder perspective. *European Sport Management Quarterly*, 9(2), 187–208.

Lyne, M., & Galloway, A. (2012). Implementation of effective alcohol control strategies is needed at large sports and entertainment events. *Australian and New Zealand Journal of Public Health*, 36(1), 55–60.

Mazanov, J., & McDermott, V. (2009). The case for a social science of drugs in sport. *Sport in Society*, 12(3), 276–295.

Mazanov, J., Hemphill, D., Connor, J., Quirk, F., & Backhouse, S. H. (2015). Australian athlete support personnel lived experience of anti-doping. *Sport Management Review*, 18(2), 218–230.

McDermott, V. (2016). *The War on Drugs in Sport: Moral Panics and Organizational Legitimacy*. Abingdon: Routledge.

Mentha, R., & Wakerman, J. (2009). An evaluation of the Australian Football League Central Australian responsible alcohol strategy 2005–07. *Health Promotion Journal of Australia*, 20(3), 208–213.

Palmer, C. (2011). Key themes and research agendas in the sport-alcohol nexus. *Journal of Sport and Social Issues*, 35(2), 168–185.

Paoli, L., & Donati, A. (2014). *The Sports Doping Market*. New York: Springer.

Petróczi, A., Taylor, G., & Naughton, D. P. (2011). Mission impossible? Regulatory and enforcement issues to ensure safety of dietary supplements. *Food and Chemical Toxicology*, 49(2), 393–402.

Pitsch, W. (2009). 'The science of doping' revisited: Fallacies of the current anti-doping regime. *European Journal of Sport Science*, 9(2), 87–95.

Pomeranz, J. L., Munsell, C. R., & Harris, J. L. (2013). Energy drinks: an emerging public health hazard for youth. *Journal of Public Health Policy*, 34(2), 254–271.

Rabin, O. (2011). Involvement of the health industry in the fight against doping in sport. *Forensic Science International*, 213(1), 10–14.

Seear, K., & Fraser, S. (2010). The 'sorry addict': Ben Cousins and the construction of drug use and addiction in elite sport. *Health Sociology Review, 19*(2), 176–191.

Sharpe, K. (2009). The economics of drugs in sport. *Sport in society, 12*(3), 344–355.

Smith, A., Stavros, C., Westberg, K., Wilson, B., & Boyle, C. (2013). Alcohol-related player behavioural transgressions: Incidences, fan media responses, and a harm-reduction alternative. *International Review for the Sociology of Sport, 49*(3–4), 400–416.

Spengler, J. O., Connaughton, D. P., & Pittman, A. T. (2006). *Risk Management in Sport and Recreation.* Champaign, IL: Human Kinetics.

Starr, R. R. (2015). Too little, too late: Ineffective regulation of dietary supplements in the United States. *American Journal of Public Health, 105*(3), 478–485.

Stewart, B., Adair, D., & Smith, A. (2011). Drivers of illicit drug use regulation in Australian sport. *Sport Management Review, 14*(3), 237–245.

Verstraete, A. (Ed.). (2011). *Workplace Drug Testing.* London, UK: Pharmaceutical Press.

Waddington, I., Christiansen, A. V., Gleaves, J., Hoberman, J., & Møller, V. (2013). Recreational drug use and sport: Time for a WADA rethink? *Performance Enhancement and Health, 2*(2), 41–47.

Chapter 9

Human resources and drugs in sport

Developing human resources to address integrity concerns arising from drugs in sport represents a significant and ongoing challenge for sports managers. Conventional thinking on the interaction between integrity management and human resource management (HRM) tends to concentrate on individual behaviour. These front line HRM responses to integrity typically include some combination of referral to managers to make integrity judgements, employing people deemed to have integrity and promoting Codes of Conduct (e.g. Jamali & El Dirani, 2013). Experience with integrity management in the public sector suggests that individually focused HRM activity needs to be supported by broader integrity systems (Six & Lawton, 2013). Such systems can be developed by considering how HRM can improve integrity management in sport by drawing on work linking corporate social responsibility (CSR) with strategic HRM (Barrena-Martinez, López-Fernández, & Romero-Fernández, 2011; Jamali, El Dirani, & Harwood, 2015; Morgeson, Aguinis, Waldman, & Siegel, 2013). The discussion of how strategic HRM can help shape responses to integrity concerns arising from managing drugs in sport examines the roles of collective bargaining, performance and incentive structures associated with employment contracts (athletes and support personnel), investment in education and the influence of managing drugs in sport on the integrity of professionals. As a result, HRM can make a significant contribution to integrity management and managing drugs in sport by developing systems that support behaviour consistent with rules- and values-based expectations.

Front line HRM responses to drugs in sport

Front line responses tend to deal with integrity as a function of the resources or tools available to the organisation in response to day-to-day management. When framed in terms of drug control-led integrity management, relying on the existing resources and tools can lead to vulnerabilities that have implications for sports production.

Referral to management

Conventional approaches to integrity management refer questions of integrity or ethics to managerial discretion, with a hierarchy of advice from operational or line staff, to line managers, middle managers, executive managers and senior executive managers. This might be captured in policies that require staff to refer issues that may compromise trust to their manager. The archetypal example of such a policy is where managers are called upon to be the arbiter of whether something is a legitimate gift or a bribe. The practice of managerial referral is entrenched in drug control for sport, with athlete support personnel reporting referral to a manager as their initial response to drug-related issues (Mazanov, Hemphill, Connor, Quirk, & Backhouse, 2015).

Referral is critically contingent on managers acting in the best interests of the organisation or sports programme rather than their own best interest. According to Principal–Agent theory (Laffont & Martimort, 2002), this occurs when the incentive structures for the manager create a moral hazard such that they stand to lose more by acting in a self-interested way. While this can be straightforward in some ways (e.g. termination clause for doping), it is less straightforward in others (e.g. protecting a programme from negative press associated with overconsumption of an alcohol sponsor's products). This can be complicated by sports managers having to balance the need to protect their programme (organisational governance) relative to protecting the integrity of sport (systemic governance). Managerial referral for matters of integrity therefore raises a potential conflict of interest (see Chapter 7), whether personal (e.g. bonus payments), professional (e.g. protecting jobs in the programme) or sectoral (e.g. protecting sport at the expense of an individual programme). While this dilemma is no different to any other market sector, it remains a fundamental challenge for HR policy relying on referral to managers where matters of integrity arise. This comes to the essence of the trust relationship that underpins integrity management; to some degree, organisations are forced to trust that managers behave in ways that preserve or enhance organisational integrity (Schein, 2010).

With the requirement to trust managers, referral then assumes that managers have some combination of experience and/or education to handle decisions with regards to integrity; that is, they are competent to make integrity-related judgements. Like the amateur traditions among athletes, the traditions of sports management have their roots in volunteers working in 'kitchen cabinets' (see Chapter 7). This tradition continued through the professionalisation of sport in the late twentieth century, with managers often drawn from within the sector (e.g. former athletes, former coaches or career administrators). Even with the rise of sports management degrees, those with such qualifications are still expected to develop breadth of experience in operational positions before being considered for managerial positions in sport (Emery, Crabtree, & Kerr, 2012). This implies that managers rely on having witnessed or been involved in enough integrity decisions to have developed heuristics of how integrity needs to be managed. As a result, managerial competence in terms of integrity in sport tends to emphasise experience over education. This may be one of the reasons underlying suggestions that the level of ethical awareness among sports managers is in need of improvement (Pritchard, 2013).

The reliance on experience extends from an assumption that greater experience leads to better ethical judgement. Unfortunately the evidence indicates that this correlation is, at best, uncertain (see Dane & Sonenshein, 2015, p. 75). This finding is complicated by evidence that athlete experience with and education about drug control for sport creates more tolerant attitudes towards drug use in sport that contrast with the prevailing anti-doping policy (Elbe & Brand, 2016; Mazanov & Huybers, 2016; Vangrunderbeek & Tolleneer, 2011). When it comes to drug control for sport, it seems that experience may lead to decisions that depart from rules- and values-based expectations among producers and consumers. As a result, relying on managerial experience to determine how best to handle integrity may be operationally expedient, but may mean sports programmes are vulnerable to integrity threats.

Hiring people with integrity

There is a standing assumption of a reciprocal relationship between personal ethics and the level of integrity within an organisation; 'good organisations' need to have 'good people' (Pritchard, 2013; Pritchard & Burton, 2014). On this logic, recruiting people on the basis of integrity should lead to higher standards of integrity within the organisation. For HRM this means hiring staff on the basis of some kind of integrity testing.

Selection processes aim to predict who is more or less likely to violate established understandings of integrity in sport. Integrity testing has become a prominent predictor in personnel selection (Van Iddekinge, Roth, Raymark, & Odle-Dusseau, 2012). Such testing typically asks respondents to self-report attitudes to and/or intentions about integrity, reveal past dishonesty, or infers risk for counter-productive workplace behaviour from combinations of individual differences (e.g. vulnerability to peer pressure). Meta-analytic evidence suggests the predictive validity of integrity testing is 'quite modest' (p. 520).

An alternative to standard integrity testing is moral disengagement. This construct seeks to explain when goals are achieved by disengaging moral restraints and minimising self-reproach for actions (Boardley & Kavussanu, 2007, p. 625). Moral disengagement in sport has typically been applied to prosocial and antisocial behaviour among athletes (e.g. Boardley

& Kavussanu, 2009) and is mainly applied to predicting athlete vulnerability to doping (see Kavussanu, 2016). While moral disengagement shows promise as a way of selecting personnel relative to integrity (Moore, Detert, Klebe Treviño, Baker, & Mayer, 2012), the predictive validity of moral disengagement as a selection tool, especially among sports managers and other athlete support personnel, is yet to be established. These results suggest that it is difficult to identify 'good people' prospectively.

Beyond integrity testing, a significant level of effort has gone into predicting athlete use of licit drugs (especially alcohol), nutritional supplements (Dietz *et al.*, 2014), illicit drugs (Dunn & Thomas, 2012) and doping (see Ntoumanis, Ng, Barkoukis, & Backhouse, 2014). The variability in what drives different drug use behaviours makes it difficult to establish a profile that could be used to select athletes likely to pattern their drug consumption to be consistent with the rules- and values-based expectations of sports production. That is, it is impossible to prospectively predict and therefore recruit athletes likely to run into problems with drugs.

Codes of conduct

Recruitment activity is often complemented with staff training in relation to Codes of Conduct. Codes of Conduct are seen as a core way of expressing an organisation's understanding of CSR. Such Codes of Conduct are typically statements outlining values that form a set of heuristics to guide both decision making and assessment of decisions. Strong Codes of Conduct are characterised as having a combination of clarity, effective promotion and effective enforcement (see Payne & Dimanche, 1996). Organisations with strong Codes of Conduct demonstrate more ethical behaviour and have more positive public perceptions of integrity (Erwin, 2011). However, Curtis and Williams (2014) report evidence that training staff about Codes of Conduct may have the opposite effect to that intended; that is, increasing awareness of unethical behaviour appears to decrease the intention to report that behaviour.

The World Anti-Doping Code's Spirit of Sport statement introduced in Chapters 4 and 6 could be thought of as the Code of Conduct for sport generally, and for drug control-led integrity management of sport specifically. To be a strong Code of Conduct that leads to more ethical behaviour and positive public perceptions of integrity, the Spirit statement needs to be clear, promoted effectively and effectively enforced. As argued in Chapter 6, ambiguity in the Spirit statement makes it vulnerable to exploitation; it fails the test of clarity. The problem of clarity is compounded with drug education programmes in sport focusing on promoting the mechanics of athlete compliance with the World Anti-Doping Code rather than discussing integrity more broadly (Mazanov *et al.*, 2015). That is, the promotion of sports 'drugs Code of Conduct' is ineffectively promoted (also, see below). Enforcement runs into two problems. The first relates to the extant difficulties of enforcement, with perceptions that athletes who dope get away with it (Gucciardi, Jalleh, & Donovan, 2011; Overbye, 2016). The second is that it appears drug control is considered a secondary or tertiary consideration in sporting practice (see Chapter 7). Where strong Codes of Conduct are characterised by clarity, promotion and enforcement, the Spirit statement is a weak Code of Conduct for managing drugs in sport. Further, if Curtis and Williams' (2014) results generalise to sport, training around the Spirit statement as a Code of Conduct for drugs in sport may make it easier to conceal the behaviour. Complementing recruitment of 'good people' with Code of Conduct training for existing staff is therefore unlikely to assist drug control-led integrity management for sport.

Beyond front line HRM

None of the three standard integrity responses from HRM appear to do much in terms of drug control for sport. Relying on managerial judgement leaves organisations vulnerable to integrity threats, especially when the manager is either driving or complicit in the arrangements (as occurred in international athletics; Pound, McLaren, & Younger, 2015). It is difficult to prospectively identify either athletes or support personnel in terms of integrity testing. Training staff relative to Codes of Conduct in relation to drug control for sport is unlikely to have the desired effect, and may lead to counterintuitive increases in undesirable behaviour. These outcomes suggest thinking about how HRM contributes to drug control-led integrity management for sport in different ways is worth examining.

CSR, strategic HRM and drugs in sport

Where CSR examines the obligations of organisations to society at large, the examination of HRM using CSR principles asks questions about the obligations to employees. This means that organisations pursuing a CSR agenda aim to provide employment conditions that go beyond legislated minima. When it comes to managing drugs in sport, this is taken to mean protecting the integrity of employees around issues of drug control. Such protection is discussed relative to collective bargaining, performance and incentives, education and the responsibility for sports managers to protect the integrity of professions working in sport from drugs.

Collective bargaining and drug control

As observed in Chapters 3 and 7, professional sport in the United States gives an indication of how collective bargaining shapes drug control-led integrity management for sport. Collective bargaining agreements on drug control for professional sports make a distinction between drug prevention and drug treatment. The former tends to be reserved for drugs typically identified under the Prohibited List. The latter tends to relate to illicit drugs or drugs of abuse (e.g. abuse of prescription drugs). Drugs of abuse trigger a treatment response rather than immediate sanction, although failure to recover from drug abuse can lead to de-registration. Such treatment approaches have had some success. The Australian Football League 'three strike' illicit drugs policy means players can test positive for illicit drugs three times, receiving treatment in response to those drug tests. On the third test, the player may be fined AU$5,000 and/or be suspended for up to 18 months. This approach to illicit drug control in sport has been successful (Harcourt, Unglik, & Cook, 2012), overcoming some of the dangers of drug exploitation arising from power differentials between leagues and athletes (Bennett, 2013).

By comparison, the anti-doping policy denies athletes the opportunity to collectively bargain the same way through the exclusion of athletes from decision-making governance (see Chapter 7). Employment contracts and membership agreements translate the anti-doping architecture from the institutional to the individual. For example, members of sports organisations (including managers, lawyers, coaches, athletes and volunteers) agree to be World Anti-Doping Code compliant either as a function of their employment contract or membership of a sports organisation. There is no room for negotiation in this clause. The consumption of drugs outside the World Anti-Doping Code can be negotiated, although this can get messy with the World Anti-Doping Code potentially covering all types of drugs (see Chapter 2).

Given there is no capacity to negotiate drug control under the World Anti-Doping Code, athlete unions have been focusing their attention on revisions to the anti-doping policy. For example, the international athlete union UNI World Athletes (formerly UNI Sport Pro) has systematically lobbied on drugs in sport issues on behalf of its more than 100,000 members, mainly to modify the anti-doping policy (Schwab, 2015). The claims point to the ineffectiveness of anti-doping as a method of drug control for sport and the hegemonic privilege granted to the policy leading to poor management practices. Predictably, a core claim within this is that anti-doping represents the vested interests of sports institutions rather than those of athletes and support personnel (see Chapter 7). Equally predictable in this institution-and-union game is that WADA can claim collective bargaining as entrenched in the processes underlying the regular review and updating of the World Anti-Doping Code, demonstrated by the extensive consultation processes behind revisions. Of course, athletes will continue to have no voice in drug control until such institutional posturing is resolved.

Despite athlete unions and sporting institutions being at an impasse when it comes to drug control, the experience with collectively bargained sports drug control in the United States shows that effective management systems can emerge without oversight from a hegemonic institution. This suggests that collectively bargained sports drug control may be one way to develop new approaches (see Chapter 4) that reflect the interests of stakeholders rather than the anti-doping duumvirate (see Chapter 7).

Performance and incentives

Employment contracts in sport often come with incentive systems designed to promote desirable outcomes. While nuanced approaches to performance measurement in sport exist (Shibli, De Bosscher, Van Bottenburg, & Westerbeek, 2013), performance used for the purposes of incentives is usually measured relative to 'performance outputs', such as the number of medals won, the number of finals berths achieved, or volume of appearances in a season. Athletes and support personnel are motivated to achieve these measurable performance outputs with short- or long-term rewards (e.g. bonuses), or relational rewards such as career development opportunities (e.g. opportunities to work in the sports media industry) (Aguinis, 2013). Like any incentive system, rational actors quickly learn to be more concerned with the achievement of the measurable output ('meeting the measure' or 'gaming the system') rather than going through the underlying process assumed to be captured by the output (see Sam & Macris, 2014, p. 514). As a result, the measurable output may lead to unintended or perverse consequences that can have profound implications for those attempting to manage integrity in sport.

Athletes

Athletes may get bonuses for winning a final, achieving a spot in a finals series or the number of games played in a season. These bonuses can lead to athletes taking a range of drugs. Performance incentives can lead to patterned drug misuse or abuse in preparation for key competitions. For example, an athlete may be so nervous before an event they are prescribed relaxants to ensure they are rested (e.g. sleeping tablets), and then prescribed stimulants to overcome the effects of the relaxant (Morse, 2013). Such patterned drug consumption could lead to dependence disorders that have significant effects well into the athlete's future, as demonstrated by the misuse and abuse of prescription sleeping pills among elite swimmers (Dunn, 2014). Performance incentives can also have a significant impact on doping, with promotion (e.g. getting a bonus) or demotion (e.g. losing a bonus) identified as motivators for doping (Mazanov, Huybers, & Connor, 2011). The corollary is that athletes some distance away from a performance threshold are unlikely to be motivated to dope.

Appearance incentives have three effects. The first is that athletes may be more likely to consume drugs in an attempt to prevent injury or illness (Mazanov, Petróczi, Bingham, & Holloway, 2008; Petróczi, Naughton, Mazanov, Holloway, & Bingham, 2007). The second is that athletes may be more likely to consume drugs to manage injury (e.g. painkilling drugs) that enable appearances (e.g. continuation in an event or early return) even though there may be longer term health implications (see Orchard, Steet, Massey, Dan, Gardiner, & Ibrahimm, 2010). The third is that, like other employees, athletes may conceal a condition and/or self-medicate in order to cope with appearance incentives. Much like other employees, athletes may turn to alcohol, prescription drugs or marijuana to self-medicate or cope with high-intensity workloads (see Chan, Johnson, Hiatt, Chou, & da Silva Cardoso, 2012). Self-medicating can also extend to responding to increases in appearance requirements, such as extensions of seasons or increases in the number of events in a programme. For example, Australian Rugby League player Andrew Johns concealed and self-medicated bipolar depression throughout his playing career, consuming a range of illicit drugs to cope with the condition, exacerbated by appearance demands (Mazanov, 2010).

Athlete support personnel

Athlete support personnel employment contracts can also include bonuses or renewal conditions predicated on managers or coaches achieving performance criteria (e.g. percentage of wins in a season, medals or finals appearances). For example, career winning percentage is a strong predictor of total compensation (including bonuses) for coaches in the Football Bowl Subdivision of the National Collegiate Athletics Association (Inoue, Plehn-Dujowich, Kent, & Swanson, 2013). The focus on performance metrics can lead support personnel to act in the best interests of their performance measures rather than, for example, the welfare of the athlete. For example, coaches may influence athletes to use drugs with demands to compete on pain medication, or make a premature return from injury, supplying illicit drugs to athletes, or setting performance criteria that can only be met using drugs (e.g. weight loss or weight gain). Away from competition, marketing officers looking to meet targets may pressure athletes to appear at sponsored events without regard for either physical or psychological recovery, leading to athlete self-medication (e.g. stimulants) or coping with related drug use (e.g. alcohol and illicit drugs) argued above. Finally, coaches remain an influence in athlete doping despite the risk of sanctions for both coaches and athletes (e.g. Huybers & Mazanov, 2012; Kirby, Moran, & Guerin, 2011; Pappa & Kennedy, 2013).

Changing definitions of performance and incentives

While the above reflects standard athlete drug-exploitation arguments (see Connor, 2009), it extends the argument by suggesting employment contracts can also drive drug consumption in sport. This means that HRM can redesign employment contracts with measurements of performance and incentives that promote functional rather than dysfunctional drug consumption. For example, rather than focusing on performance outputs, employment contracts could look to include a more graduated approach based on the more nuanced understanding of sports performance offered by Shibli *et al.* (2013) via incentives for throughputs (production processes) and qualification outputs (achieving performance milestones). However, imposing ever smaller increments of performance and incentives leads to undesirable inflation of bureaucracy and associated transaction costs (Sam & Macris, 2014). Put simply, such an approach increases costs.

Another approach is to measure and incentivise different behaviours using positive (reward) and negative reinforcement (withdrawal of reward). This approach stands in contrast to the extensive analysis on the role of punishment in sports drug control (Dilger, Frick, & Tolsdorf, 2007; Maennig, 2002; Kirstein, 2014). For example, Mazanov *et al.* (2011) argue the impact of promotion or demotion could be moderated with standardised salaries for athletes and incentive payments held in trust payable upon retirement from sport (a deferred compensation model; Maennig, 2009). Individual and group incentives might be introduced in regards to drug behaviour that promotes certain types of drug consumption (e.g. consultation with health professionals) and dissuades other types of consumption (e.g. athletes stop each other from binging on alcohol or risk losing a group bonus). Athlete welfare in regards to drugs may be enhanced by introducing maximum as well as minimum numbers of appearances in a season (see Aubel & Ohl, 2014, Proposition 2). Incentives could be moderated based on injury volume or re-injury rates, such that athletes and coaches become more conservative about returns from injury.

A closer look at how performance measurement and incentives influence drug behaviour in sport suggests that HRM can have a significant impact. Employment contracts can be designed around principles that encourage desirable drug behaviour and discourage undesirable behaviour. Incentives can also be designed to promote internal monitoring (e.g. athletes and support personnel regulating each other's behaviour) rather than external monitoring (e.g. WADA or the media).

Drug education

Drug education in sport has become increasingly synonymous with educating athletes and support personnel about athlete compliance with the

World Anti-Doping Code, rather than educating athletes about the role and implications of drugs in sport more broadly (alcohol education being a possible exception). HRM has focused on anti-doping education rather than other forms of drug education for both strategic and operational reasons.

Strategically, systemic governance mechanisms (see Chapter 7) make World Anti-Doping Code compliance status and therefore access to sport contingent upon signatories offering anti-doping education (Article 18.1). This makes the decision of where to invest scarce resources across the spectrum of personnel management activities (e.g. talent identification, recruitment, professional development and career transitions), relatively straightforward. Failure to comply with the World Anti-Doping Code means denial of access to sport whereas a failure to educate athletes about alcohol abuse can be managed reactively (see Chapters 5 and 8). The rational response is therefore to invest in anti-doping education to ensure World Anti-Doping Code compliance and preserve access to sporting events, while investment in other forms of drug education can be made when the need becomes apparent. The overwhelming focus on anti-doping education has put sport at risk of failing to adequately address education for other drugs (Kondric et al., 2011).

Operationally, the interest in promoting anti-doping education emerges when considering the risk key personnel could be lost to a sports programme as a result of either intentional or inadvertent ADRVs. For example, the team sports physician could be prohibited immediately before an event, with clinical handover to a new physician prevented under Article 2.10 (association with a person under a sanction). Equally, an athlete might be unexpectedly lost to a programme having failed to be at the nominated location for out-of-competition drug testing. As a result, HRM has good reasons for focusing on anti-doping education over other forms of drug education.

Despite the focus and investment in anti-doping education, evidence suggests the investment in anti-doping education is insufficient to help athletes and support personnel comply with the World Anti-Doping Code. The level of knowledge among athletes and support personnel is best characterised as ignorance. Athletes from all levels of sport have shown a basic lack of awareness (Backhouse, McKenna, Robinson, & Atkin, 2007). While this appears to be improving, athletes are still at risk of ADRV because they fail to understand their obligations (Morente-Sánchez & Zabala, 2013). A similar pattern is repeated among support personnel (Mazanov, Backhouse, Connor, Hemphill, & Quirk, 2014). While medical practitioners have the best knowledge about anti-doping across support personnel (Mazanov et al., 2014), the level of knowledge they have is still insufficient to avoid committing ADRVs (Backhouse & McKenna, 2011). This combination of results indicates that other support personnel, such as coaches, sports trainers, psychologists and administrators, lack sufficient knowledge to support World Anti-Doping Code compliance.

An unexpected issue for HRM is that, like staff training on Codes of Conduct, education about anti-doping appears to increase the likelihood of doping. Athletes who demonstrate an understanding of the World Anti-Doping Code are more likely to consume performance enhancing nutritional supplements (Mazanov et al., 2008) and to dope (Loraschi, Galli, & Consentino, 2014; Ntoumanis et al., 2014). Given evidence of a correlation between consuming performance enhancing drugs and increased risk of abusing licit (e.g. alcohol) and illicit drugs (e.g. marijuana and hallucinogens) (Laure & Binsinger, 2007; Yusko, Buckman, White, & Pandina, 2008), anti-doping education could paradoxically lead athletes to use, misuse or abuse drugs in ways that violate rules- and values-based expectations.

The evidence suggests that integrity management for sport needs drug education rather than anti-doping education. The correlation between doping and other drug consumption indicates that using drug education in sport as part of integrity management initiatives should never be about a single type of drug. Rather than mitigating integrity risks, the myopic focus on anti-doping education (Kondric et al., 2011) appears to make sport more vulnerable to integrity violations associated with drug use, misuse and abuse.

Professional integrity

Drug control for sport extends to managing the integrity of professionals practising in sport (e.g. medical practitioners, lawyers and psychologists). If sport wants to compete with other market sectors looking to attract and retain professionals (e.g. the military), it needs to ensure that managing integrity for sport is sympathetic with the maintenance of integrity in allied market sectors. For example, there is evidence to suggest the anti-doping policy is discouraging medical experts from engaging with sport (Fincouer, van de Ven, & Mulrooney, 2015). HRM has responsibility for the maintenance of professional integrity in two ways. The first is protecting the integrity of professionals in sport from so-called 'rogue scientists'. The second is a dilemma that emerges from protecting the integrity of professionals working in sport.

Rogue scientists

Sports programmes receive unsolicited offers from both legitimately qualified professionals and proverbial 'rogue scientists' with claims their drug-based innovations provide competitive advantage (from injury recovery to performance enhancement). The Australian Senate (2013) identified that the sports sector needed to protect itself from rogue scientists or face increased regulation in the space. The challenge for HRM is discriminating between entrepreneurs that help and rogues that harm a sports programme.

The immediate answer is to draw on in-house expertise to assess the claims made by the prospective professional (assuming in-house expertise also acts in the best interests of the programme; see Chapter 7). This investment of resources in assessing offers indicates some selection routine is needed, the effectiveness of which varies by the volume of offers administered. Low volumes of offers can probably be managed in-house at relatively low cost to the programme. High volumes of offers, like any selection protocol, compel administrative architecture to separate claims, such as redeploying in-house expertise (e.g. review by coaching and medical staff) or outsourcing. Programmes without in-house expertise and few resources may have to rely on staff donating time to develop the expertise necessary to respond to offers, or rely on better-resourced sports programmes sharing expertise and experience. The costs associated with either approach indicate a market signal is needed to enable a more efficient method of discrimination between legitimate professionals and rogue scientists.

The market signal can be achieved in two ways. The first is accreditation. The Australian Senate (2013) raised concerns too few people qualified as accredited sports scientists, leading to a proliferation of people claiming expertise in the area without oversight. The Senate recommendations sent a blunt warning that accreditation needed to be resolved or regulation would be imposed in the form of 'sports scientist' becoming a registered health profession (alongside dentistry, medicine, nursing, psychology and podiatry). The second is a market driven mechanism, such as setting up a reputation driven database (e.g. social media) that discriminates legitimate professionals from rogue scientists. Either approach would enable more reliable and efficient selection of legitimate professionals, and reduce the potential for drug-related violations of integrity.

Protecting the integrity of sports professionals

Protecting sports professionals from 'rogue scientists' also emerges in the form of professional practice. There are clearly some who use their professional skills to subvert drug control; for example, BALCO was a group of professionals designing and selling undetectable performance enhancing drugs. Other 'rogue scientists' may be health practitioners who see the professional obligation to protect athlete health from drug misuse and abuse through supervision as superior to drug control (see Hoff, 2012). This professional conflict is apparent in the 'disclosure dilemma' (Mazanov, 2013; McNamee & Phillips, 2011).

The essence of the dilemma emerges from reporting obligations. For example, an athlete may disclose they have used marijuana in competition to a medical practitioner seeking information to avoid contraindications. Under the World Anti-Doping Code, the medical practitioner is obliged to report the athlete for use of a drug prohibited in competition. However, the medical practitioner is also bound by a professional requirement to protect the confidentiality necessary to ensure trust in the doctor–patient relationship. Equally, an athlete may disclose doping to a lawyer as part of contract negotiations; it is uncertain how legal privilege applies in this context (Rule of Law Institute of Australia, 2013). In working to preserve the integrity of sport the World Anti-Doping Code may diminish the integrity of professionals working in sport.

Rational responses to the dilemma create perverse incentives for both athletes and support personnel. Athletes would be justifiably reluctant to disclose information about their drug use for fear of sanction, leading to gaps in information necessary to manage the athlete. For example, an athlete with Anabolic Steroid Dependence Disorder may hesitate to seek support in overcoming their dependence. The longer term implications are that athletes may no longer trust professional advice as a result of being reported, and come to rely on advice from practitioners without a professional background (e.g. medical advice from trainers). Professionals who report drug using athletes risk destroying the trust relationship with athletes, their professional reputation and livelihood through deregistration for breaching confidentiality, or risk being banned from sport (and potentially their livelihood) for failure to report. In both instances, the attempt to preserve the integrity of sport creates incentives towards a 'don't ask, don't tell' approach that potentially compromises both the availability of the athlete and support personnel.

Professionals only add value to sports programmes when they are able to practise their profession. As a consequence, HRM needs to find a way to ensure that professionals can practise their profession within sport to add that value. For example, it may be appropriate for HRM to negotiate the relationship between sport and professional obligations on behalf of professionals working in sport. This may involve drawing together professional associations (e.g. the American College of Sports Medicine) with organisations who manage registration (e.g. State Medical Licensing Boards) with sports to resolve this question. In doing so, it needs to be made clear whether licensed medical professionals are at risk of losing their licence to practice for disclosing ADRV. While such an approach would be consistent with other exceptions to client confidentiality (e.g. threatening murder), it raises questions of proportionality in terms of whether athlete drug consumption is a significant enough threat to warrant being made such an exception. The alternative is that professional privilege is protected, putting the welfare of the athlete above that of drug control. Doing so begins to point towards a harm-minimisation approach to drug control for sport argued in Chapter 4.

Integrity and sports professionals

Attracting and retaining professionals can add value to sport. Sport needs to maintain the integrity of its relationship with such professionals, or risk losing them to other market sectors in need of their expertise (e.g. veteran rehabilitation). This can be achieved by ensuring sport is a place where professionals can practise in ways that are consistent with their professional ethics, without the interference of rogue elements besmirching the role of professionals in sport.

Linking CSR and the HRM of drugs in sport

The stage is now set to move beyond the standard front line responses towards a deeper consideration of how HRM can contribute to drug control-led integrity management for sport. Indeed, sport could expand its status as a fertile ground for testing new ideas to consider how strategic HRM can inform CSR practices (Barrena-Martinez *et al.*, 2011; Jamali *et al.*, 2015). In particular, sport has the capacity to inform the dynamic and reciprocal interaction between HRM and CSR, such as the relationship between integrity in sport and integrity in the professions (e.g. medicine). A better understanding of these synergies may also inform the effort to manage employment conditions, through collective bargaining, incentives and education, thought to drive CSR (Barrena-Martinez *et al.*, 2011). Thus, it seems that the effort to use HRM to develop drug control-led integrity for sport also has an important role in developing the practice and evaluation of the impact strategic HRM has in relation to the CSR agenda.

References

Aguinis, H. (2013). *Performance Management* (3rd Ed.). Essex: Pearson.

Aubel, O., & Ohl, F. (2014). An alternative approach to the prevention of doping in cycling. *International Journal of Drug Policy*, 25(6), 1094–1102.

Australian Senate (2013). *Practice of Sports Science in Australia*. Canberra: Commonwealth of Australia.

Backhouse, S. H., & McKenna, J. (2011). Doping in sport: A review of medical practitioners' knowledge, attitudes and beliefs. *International Journal of Drug Policy*, 22(3), 198–202.

Backhouse, S., McKenna, J., Robinson, S., & Atkin, A. (2007). *International Literature Review: Attitudes, Behaviours, Knowledge and Education – Drugs in Sport: Past, present and future*. Available at: https://wada-main-prod.s3.amazonaws.com/resources/files/backhouse_et_al_full_report.pdf (accessed 27 February 2016).

Barrena-Martinez, J., López-Fernández, M., & Romero-Fernández, P. M. (2011). Research proposal on the relationship between corporate social responsibility and strategic human resource management. *International Journal of Management and Enterprise Development*, 10(2–3), 173–187.

Bennett, D. (2013). Harm reduction and NFL drug policy. *Journal of Sport and Social Issues*, *37*(2), 160–175.

Boardley, I. D., & Kavussanu, M. (2007). Development and validation of the moral disengagement in sport scale. *Journal of Sport and Exercise Psychology*, *29*(5), 608–628.

Boardley, I. D., & Kavussanu, M. (2009). The influence of social variables and moral disengagement on prosocial and antisocial behaviours in field hockey and netball. *Journal of Sports Sciences*, *27*(8), 843–854.

Chan, F., Johnson, E., Hiatt, E. K., Chou, C. C., & da Silva Cardoso, E. (2012). Self-medication and illicit drug use in the workplace. In R. Gatchel, & I. Schultz (Eds.), *Handbook of Occupational Health and Wellness* (pp. 201–218). New York: Springer US.

Connor, J. (2009). The athlete as widget: How exploitation explains elite sport. *Sport in Society*, *12*(10), 1369–1377.

Curtis, M. B., & Williams, J. M. (2014). The impact of culture and training on code of conduct effectiveness: Reporting of observed unethical behavior. In C. Jeffrey (Ed.), *Research on Professional Responsibility and Ethics in Accounting (Volume 18)* (pp. 1–31). Bingley, UK: Emerald.

Dane, E., & Sonenshein, S. (2015). On the role of experience in ethical decision making at work: An ethical expertise perspective. *Organizational Psychology Review*, *5*(1), 74–96.

Dietz, P., Ulrich, R., Niess, A., Best, R., Simon, P., & Striegel, H. (2014). Prediction profiles for nutritional supplement use among young German elite athletes. *International Journal of Sport Nutrition and Exercise Metabolism*, *24*(6), 623–631.

Dilger, A., Frick, B., & Tolsdorf, F. (2007). Are athletes doped? Some theoretical arguments and empirical evidence. *Contemporary Economic Policy*, *25*(4), 604–615.

Dunn, M. (2014). The importance of understanding motives for prescription substance use and misuse in sport. *Performance Enhancement and Health*, *3*(2), 102–104.

Dunn, M., & Thomas, J. O. (2012). A risk profile of elite Australian athletes who use illicit drugs. *Addictive Behaviors*, *37*(1), 144–147.

Elbe, A. M., & Brand, R. (2016). The effect of an ethical decision-making training on young athletes' attitudes toward doping. *Ethics and Behavior*, *26*(1), 32–44.

Emery, P. R., Crabtree, R. M., & Kerr, A. K. (2012). The Australian sport management job market: An advertisement audit of employer need. *Annals of Leisure Research*, *15*(4), 335–353.

Erwin, P. M. (2011). Corporate codes of conduct: The effects of code content and quality on ethical performance. *Journal of Business Ethics*, *99*(4), 535–548.

Fincoeur, B., van de Ven, K., & Mulrooney, K. J. (2015). The symbiotic evolution of anti-doping and supply chains of doping substances: How criminal networks may benefit from anti-doping policy. *Trends in Organized Crime*, *18*(3), 229–250.

Gucciardi, D. F., Jalleh, G., & Donovan, R. J. (2011). An examination of the Sport Drug Control Model with elite Australian athletes. *Journal of Science and Medicine in Sport*, *14*(6), 469–476.

Harcourt, P. R., Unglik, H., & Cook, J. L. (2012). A strategy to reduce illicit drug use is effective in elite Australian football. *British Journal of Sports Medicine*, 46(13), 943–945.

Hoff, D. (2012). Doping, risk and abuse: An interview study of elite athletes with a history of steroid use. *Performance Enhancement and Health*, 1(2), 61–65.

Huybers, T., & Mazanov, J. (2012). What would Kim do: A choice study of projected athlete doping considerations. *Journal of Sport Management*, 26(4), 322–334.

Inoue, Y., Plehn-Dujowich, J. M., Kent, A., & Swanson, S. (2013). Roles of performance and human capital in college football coaches' compensation. *Journal of Sport Management*, 27(1), 73–83.

Jamali, D., & El Dirani, A. (2013). CSR and HRM for workplace integrity: Advancing the business ethics agenda. In W. Amann, & A. Stachowicz-Stanusch (Eds.), *Integrity in Organizations: Building the Foundations for Humanistic Management* (pp. 439–456). Houndmills, UK: Palgrave Macmillan.

Jamali, D. R., El Dirani, A. M., & Harwood, I. A. (2015). Exploring human resource management roles in corporate social responsibility: The CSR-HRM co-creation model. *Business Ethics: A European Review*, 24(2), 125–143.

Kavussanu, M. (2016). Moral disengagement and doping. In V. Barkoukis, L. Lazarus, & H. Tsorbatzoudis (Eds.), *The Psychology of Doping in Sport* (pp. 151–164). Abingdon: Routledge.

Kirby, K., Moran, A., & Guerin, S. (2011). A qualitative analysis of the experiences of elite athletes who have admitted to doping for performance enhancement. *International Journal of Sport Policy and Politics*, 3(2), 205–224.

Kirstein, R. (2014). Doping, the inspection game, and Bayesian enforcement. *Journal of Sports Economics*, 15(4), 385–409.

Kondric, M., Sekulic, D., Petróczi, A., Ostojic, L., Rodek, J., & Ostojic, Z. (2011). Is there a danger for myopia in anti-doping education? Comparative analysis of substance use and misuse in Olympic racket sports calls for a broader approach. *Substance Abuse Treatment, Prevention and Policy*, 6(27).

Laffont, J. J., & Martimort, D. (2002). *The Theory of Incentives: The Principal–Agent Model*. Princeton, NJ: Princeton University Press.

Laure, P., & Binsinger, C. (2007). Doping prevalence among preadolescent athletes: A 4-year follow-up. *British Journal of Sports Medicine*, 41(10), 660–663.

Loraschi, A., Galli, N., & Cosentino, M. (2014). Dietary supplement and drug use and doping knowledge and attitudes in Italian young elite cyclists. *Clinical Journal of Sport Medicine*, 24(3), 238–244.

Maennig, W. (2002). On the economics of doping and corruption in international sports. *Journal of Sports Economics*, 3(1), 61–89.

Maennig, W. (2009). Pecuniary disincentives in the anti-doping fight. *Economic Analysis and Policy*, 39(3), 349.

Mazanov, J. (2010). Drug use and abuse by athletes. In S. J. Hanrahan, & M. B. Anderson (Eds.), *Routledge Handbook of Applied Sport Psychology* (pp. 214–223). Abingdon: Routledge.

Mazanov, J. (2013). The management of performance enhancing drugs in high performance sport. In P. Sotiriadou, & V. De Bossche (Eds.), *Managing High Performance Sport* (pp. 272–294). Abingdon: Routledge.

Mazanov, J., Petróczi, A., Bingham, J., & Holloway, A. (2008). Towards an empirical model of performance enhancing supplement use: a pilot study among high performance UK athletes. *Journal of Science and Medicine in Sport*, *11*(2), 185–190.

Mazanov, J., & Huybers, T. (2016). Societal and athletes' perspectives on doping use in sport: The Spirit of Sport. In V. Barkoukis, L. Lazarus, & H. Tsorbatzoudis (Eds.), *The Psychology of Doping in Sport* (pp. 140–150). Abingdon: Routledge.

Mazanov, J., Huybers, T., & Connor, J. (2011). Qualitative evidence of a primary intervention point for elite athlete doping. *Journal of Science and Medicine in Sport*, *14*(2), 106–110.

Mazanov, J., Petróczi, A., Bingham, J., & Holloway, A. (2008). Towards an empirical model of performance enhancing supplement use: A pilot study among high performance UK athletes. *Journal of Science and Medicine in Sport*, *11*(2), 185–190.

Mazanov, J., Backhouse, S., Connor, J., Hemphill, D., & Quirk, F. (2014). Athlete support personnel and anti-doping: Knowledge, attitudes, and ethical stance. *Scandinavian Journal of Medicine and Science in Sports*, *24*(5), 846–856.

Mazanov, J., Hemphill, D., Connor, J., Quirk, F., & Backhouse, S. H. (2015). Australian athlete support personnel lived experience of anti-doping. *Sport Management Review*, *18*(2), 218–230.

McNamee, M., & Phillips, N. (2011). Confidentiality, disclosure and doping in sports medicine. *British Journal of Sports Medicine*, *45*(3), 174–177.

Moore, C., Detert, J. R., Klebe Treviño, L., Baker, V. L., & Mayer, D. M. (2012). Why employees do bad things: Moral disengagement and unethical organizational behavior. *Personnel Psychology*, *65*(1), 1–48.

Morente-Sánchez, J., & Zabala, M. (2013). Doping in sport: a review of elite athletes' attitudes, beliefs, and knowledge. *Sports Medicine*, *43*(6), 395–411.

Morgeson, F. P., Aguinis, H., Waldman, D. A., & Siegel, D. S. (2013). Extending corporate social responsibility research to the human resource management and organizational behavior domains: A look to the future. *Personnel Psychology*, *66*(4), 805–824.

Morse, E. D. (2013). Substance use in athletes. In D. A. Baron, C. L. Reardon, & S. H. Baron (Eds.), *Clinical Sports Psychiatry: An International Perspective* (pp. 3–12). Oxford, UK: Wiley.

Ntoumanis, N., Ng, J. Y., Barkoukis, V., & Backhouse, S. (2014). Personal and psychosocial predictors of doping use in physical activity settings: A meta-analysis. *Sports Medicine*, *44*(11), 1603–1624.

Orchard, J.W., Steet, E., Massey, A., Dan, S., Gardiner, B., & Ibrahimm, A. (2010). Long-term safety of using local anaesthetic injections in professional rugby league. *American Journal of Sports Medicine* *38*(11), 2259–2266.

Overbye, M. (2016). Doping control in sport: An investigation of how elite athletes perceive and trust the functioning of the doping testing system in their sport. *Sport Management Review*, *19*(1), 6–22.

Pappa, E., & Kennedy, E. (2013). 'It was my thought … he made it a reality': Normalization and responsibility in athletes' accounts of performance-enhancing drug use. *International Review for the Sociology of Sport*, *48*(3), 277–294.

Payne, D., & Dimanche, F. (1996). Towards a code of conduct for the tourism industry: An ethics model. *Journal of Business Ethics*, *15*(9), 997–1007.

Petróczi, A., Naughton, D. P., Mazanov, J., Holloway, A., & Bingham, J. (2007). Limited agreement exists between rationale and practice in athletes' supplement use for maintenance of health: A retrospective study. *Nutrition Journal*, 6(34).

Pound, R., McLaren, R., & Younger, G. (2015). *Independent Commission Report #1*. Montreal: World Anti-Doping Agency.

Pritchard, M. P. (2013). Ethical decision making in sport and business. In M. P. Pritchard, & J. L. Stinson (Eds.), *Leveraging Brands in Sport Business* (pp. 66–86). Abingdon: Routledge.

Pritchard, M. P., & Burton, R. (2014). Ethical failures in sport business: Directions for research. *Sport Marketing Quarterly*, 23(2), 86–99.

Rule of Law Institute of Australia (2013). Australian Sports Anti-Doping Act. Available at: www.ruleoflaw.org.au/australian-sports-anti-doping-authority-act/ (accessed 27 February 2016).

Sam, M. P., & Macris, L. I. (2014). Performance regimes in sport policy: exploring consequences, vulnerabilities and politics. *International Journal of Sport Policy and Politics*, 6(3), 513–532.

Schein, E. H. (2010). *Organizational Culture and Leadership* (4th Ed.). San Francisco: John Wiley & Sons.

Schwab, B. (2015). The Global Players' and Athletes' associated for professional sport – UNI World Athletes explained. Available at: www.uniglobalunion.org/news/uni-world-athletes-new-global-players-association-professional-sport (accessed 27 February 2016).

Shibli, S., De Bosscher, V., Van Bottenburg, M., & Westerbeek, H. (2013). Measuring performance and success in elite sports. In P. Sotiriadou, & V. De Bosscher (Eds.), *Managing High Performance Sport* (pp. 30–44). Abingdon: Routledge.

Six, F., & Lawton, A. (2013). Towards a theory of integrity systems: A configurational approach. *International Review of Administrative Sciences*, 79(4), 639–658.

Van Iddekinge, C. H., Roth, P. L., Raymark, P. H., & Odle-Dusseau, H. N. (2012). The criterion-related validity of integrity tests: An updated meta-analysis. *Journal of Applied Psychology*, 97(3), 499.

Vangrunderbeek, H., & Tolleneer, J. (2011). Student attitudes towards doping in sport: Shifting from repression to tolerance? *International Review for the Sociology of Sport*, 46(3), 346–357.

Yusko, D. A., Buckman, J. F., White, H. R., & Pandina, R. J. (2008). Alcohol, tobacco, illicit drugs, and performance enhancers: A comparison of use by college student athletes and non-athletes. *Journal of American College Health*, 57(3), 281–290.

Chapter 10

Marketing, integrity management and drugs in sport

Co-authored with Dr Daniel Prior, School of Business, UNSW-Canberra

Sports have become an important marketing vehicle for many organisations. Sponsors and advertisers often seek an association with the positive characteristics of sport to boost their own brands (Funk, Alexandris, & McDonald, 2008; Wang & Kaplanidou, 2013). Accordingly, sports marketing has emerged from the general marketing literature as an important sub-discipline with its own unique characteristics and features. Despite the relationship between sport and drugs being widely understood in marketing contexts, it is a surprising omission from sports marketing texts (e.g. Chadwick, Chanavat, & Desbordes, 2016). While there is interest in the notion of customer promise management (the warrant that delivery of sports-related products and services are consistent with the rules- and values-based expectations that form the basis of the trust relationship), drugs in sport receive very little research attention from a marketing perspective (Prior, O'Reilly, Mazanov, & Huybers, 2013). The discussion of marketing, integrity management and drugs in sport therefore has value in terms of drawing together the literature on the field, but also points to where deeper consideration of the issue by sports marketing may be warranted.

Rather than attempt to address the breadth that marketing scholarship allows (e.g. consumer behaviour, brand loyalty or communications), the discussion focuses on three very different challenges for sports marketing arising from drug control-led integrity management. The first explores the issues that have emerged from the relationship sport has had with advertising and sponsorship of licit drugs, and how they inform marketing of new drugs (e.g. e-cigarettes). The second arises from the increasing difficulties sport faces in managing the integrity of the 'customer promise' in the face of drug-related scandals, usually interpreted as a form of product harm crisis management and service failure management focusing on how the organisation can recover sales in the wake of such incidents. The third challenge comes from the implications arising from the use of anti-doping as a marketing device.

Marketing of licit drugs in sport

While sport has had a longer and stronger history with alcohol, it was the relationship with tobacco that entrenched the correlation between sport and the marketing of 'sin' products (Crompton, 2014). Sin products, such as tobacco, alcohol and gambling (Davidson, 2003), look to associate themselves with sport to exploit halo effects. The halo effect refers to a psychological process where positive attribution on one dimension generalises to other dimensions (e.g. attractive people are also more intelligent and trustworthy). As a result, associating a sin product with the positive values attributed to a sports property can potentially overcome the socially undesirable product characteristics (McGhee, 2012). Such attributions include associating the positive qualities attributed to a celebrity athlete, or linking the physiologically driven emotional response to sports experiences with a drug (e.g. consuming alcohol while watching a sporting event; Meier, 2011). What is understood to be a sin product in sport appears to be a function of whether a product contradicts 'sport as health' discourses (Hanstad & Waddington, 2009; McDaniel, Mason, & Kinney, 2004), such as foods high in fat, salt or sugar (HFSS) (Crompton, 2014). This is typically framed in terms of how marketing activities (e.g. advertising during sports events) increase the likelihood of consumers engaging in discretionary health risk behaviours that contradict medical and public health discourses, including overeating HFSS foods, misusing alcohol and gambling addiction (e.g. Lindsay et al., 2013; Lamont, Hing, & Gainsbury, 2011). The classic example of using sport to market a sin product is tobacco, both for the use of halo effects in relation to sport and for contradicting the 'sport as health' discourse.

Experience with tobacco sponsorship has identified that sport is an ideal vehicle to market sin products to children (see Chapter 3). In particular, the licit drugs industry uses sport to overcome advertising regulations designed to limit children's exposure to sin products. The use of sport as a vehicle to market to children is a long established tradition (e.g. Babe Ruth's touting of tobacco products) (McGhee, 2012). Tobacco companies identified adolescence as the time to establish brand capital, as this is when drug consumption behaviour and preferences emerge (see Chapter 11). These preferences persist through to adulthood. For example, cigarette brand loyalty has remained among the highest across product categories over time (Dawes, 2014). Although tobacco was forced to exit sport with regards to combustible cigarettes, the sports marketing strategy pioneered by tobacco has been replicated with other licit drugs. It is therefore unsurprising that sport dominates alcohol sponsorship activity in the United States (Belt et al., 2014), presumably for its capacity to market alcohol to children. For example, there is evidence alcohol brand preferences persist from adolescence through to adulthood (Siegel et al., 2015), suggesting that brand capital developed through sports-related exposure converts to brand loyalty (capture) and potentially lifetime consumption. It is also unsurprising that the regulation of alcohol-related marketing activities is beginning to look a lot like the regulation that forced tobacco out of sport (Crompton, 2014).

Given sport's value in youth markets, sport has become a significant component of the marketing mix for caffeinated beverage brands (high energy drinks) aiming to secure a share of the adolescent and youth market (Emond, Sargent, & Gilbert-Diamond, 2015; Harris & Munsell, 2015). Marketing caffeine using sport also looks to exploit the 'legal' performance enhancing effect across recreational, non-elite and elite athletes (Del Coso, Lara, & López-Muñoz, 2015). As noted in Chapter 2, the proliferation in availability of caffeine products, especially in sweetened carbonated forms, has led to concerns about the long-term health implications of sustained caffeine use among adolescents generally (Sanchis-Gomar, Pareja-Galeano, Cervellin, Lippi, & Earnest, 2015) and misuse or abuse among athletes specifically (Duchan, Patel, & Feucht, 2010; Reissig, Strain, & Griffiths, 2009). The health concerns associated with this form of caffeine consumption are leading to calls for regulation (Pomeranz, Munsell, & Harris, 2013) which bear striking similarity with the calls that led to restrictions on cigarette and alcohol marketing.

At this point it is worth observing that sports' marketing has become a battleground between the private interests of licit drug companies and the public health industry. In terms of integrity management, the question of licit drugs has the potential to undermine the values-based expectations of sport as an inherently virtuous activity that promotes normatively constructed physical, psychological, social and spiritual 'health' (see Chapters 1 and 6). Put simply, the idea that sport promotes drugs that are likely to compromise health appears to be a problem (Hanstad & Waddington, 2009). However, given Australian consumers consistently rate health as a secondary consideration in what makes sport valuable (Mazanov, Huybers, & Connor, 2012), the health implications of licit drugs appear to be more of a concern for public health advocates than consumers. In fact, consumers seem comfortable with the idea that alcohol and caffeine are legitimate sponsors of sport. Just how far this comfort extends will be tested with the entry of two new 'licit' drugs to the sports marketing arena; e-cigarettes and marijuana.

E-cigarettes

The arrival of electronic nicotine delivery systems (commonly known as e-cigarettes) represents a return to nicotine inhalation that may make combusted tobacco obsolete (cigarettes). Importantly, e-cigarettes have differential regulation across markets. For example, at the time of writing, the

United Kingdom and the United States had liberal regulation, whereas Australia and Canada had more restrictive policies (Kornfield, Huang, Vera, & Emery, 2015). Importantly, the demonisation of combustible cigarette smoking meant that e-cigarettes could be classified as a sin product – which meant marketing of the product needed to overcome public health's social construction of nicotine inhalation as a socially unacceptable behaviour.

The marketing of e-cigarettes cleverly co-opted public health discourses and social marketing narratives by arguing that, like other nicotine delivery systems (e.g. patches, pills, gums and sprays), they are designed to help people quit smoking cigarettes (McKee, 2013), even though the evidence indicates the opposite is true (Kalkhoran & Glantz, 2016). Co-opting health discourses has seen e-cigarettes broadly marketed as a 'healthier' version of nicotine consumption. This has been promoted by changing how the behaviour is characterised, replacing the stigmatised term 'smoking' with 'vaping' (Fairchild, Bayer, & Colgrove, 2014). Such marketing has clearly had the desired effect, with e-cigarettes perceived to be less likely to cause disease (Pepper, Emery, Ribisl, Rini, & Brewer, 2015). While the introduction of e-cigarettes has caused something of a crisis in the medical and public health communities, there is evidence that e-cigarette vaping is a more socially acceptable form of nicotine inhalation than cigarette smoking in the United States (Trumbo & Harper, 2015). Qualitative evidence indicates that, while consumers are aware of their general lack of knowledge about e-cigarettes (health or otherwise), they are more favourably disposed towards them, captured by one focus group participant as, 'You know what? It's not smoke. It's not tar. It's not 4,000 chemicals' (Coleman *et al.*, 2016).

The marketing budgets for e-cigarette brands are increasing (Kornfield *et al.*, 2015), and sport is a growing part of the marketing mix. An examination of e-cigarette marketing in the United Kingdom revealed sponsorship of football, motor racing, powerboating and superbike racing, and distribution of free e-cigarette samples at sports events (De Andrade, Hastings, Angus, Dixon, & Purves, 2013). Their analysis of e-cigarette marketing showed that e-cigarette brands replicated strategies and tactics historically used by combustible cigarette brands, such as the replication of artwork and copy from across the history of tobacco marketing.

The essential dilemma for sport is that it risks repeating all the problems that arose from the relationship with combustible cigarette brands. While sport may enjoy significant sponsorship and advertising revenues, there is also a risk that sport may repeat the experience of attracting increasing external regulation. From a strategic point of view, sport should expect and plan for external regulation from the outset. Rather than repeating the error of having a symbiotic relationship between brands such that external regulation threatens survival (e.g. tobacco and snooker), sport needs to ensure that e-cigarettes are part of a diverse portfolio of sponsorship and advertising across sin and non-sin product categories. That is, sports need to avoid becoming sports sponsored e-cigarette events the same way some sports have become sports sponsored alcohol events (Jones, 2010).

In terms of drug control-led integrity management, sport in the United Kingdom and United States accepting sponsorship from e-cigarette brands is consistent with rules-based integrity. In terms of values-based expectations, the risk to sport appears to be less one of health (given the relative perception of e-cigarettes as 'healthier' and the disjoint between sport and health) than of breaching expectations around marketing to children. Under corporate social responsibility (CSR), sport should use its influence to ensure that children are protected from e-cigarette brand marketing activities, rather than risk repeating the failures to manage its relationship with combustible cigarettes.

Marijuana

While the challenges for marketing e-cigarettes in sport lie in overcoming a socially unacceptable licit drug, marijuana faces very different challenges as it transitions from being an illicit to a licit drug in some jurisdictions. For example, Canada has taken an increasingly tolerant approach to the medical use of marijuana since 2001 (Fischer, Kuganesan, & Room, 2015), and considerable variation in laws governing marijuana has emerged across the United States (ranging from criminal prohibition to medical use to recreational use). The liberalisation of marijuana production in Canada has raised the prospect of marijuana sponsorship of a sports team (Mallen & Mansurov, 2015).

At first blush marijuana sponsorship of sport may seem problematic, but some problems are readily resolved. For example, the contradiction between the 'great sporting myth' and the 'drugs are bad' trope that marijuana might invoke among consumers may be less relevant to a sport with an existing culture of marijuana consumption (e.g. snowboarding; Thorpe, 2012). Equally, there is no reason to expect that an athlete's willingness or refusal to endorse the sponsor's product should pose a problem (e.g. verbally or being seen to use), especially given established protocols with regards to managing endorsement refusal of alcohol by athletes on religious grounds.

However, there are some other issues that may be more difficult to overcome. Based on the experiences with other licit drugs, marketing strategies would need to address consumer concerns about health and advertising to children. There is a significant integrity risk if sport allows itself to be used to market marijuana consumption (especially smoking) to children the same way sport was used by tobacco. Further, marijuana sponsorship raises some difficult questions given its status on the in-competition Prohibited List. Marijuana sponsorship of a Canadian Olympic snowboarding squad would be an interesting and novel challenge for sports policy makers and sports managers alike.

While the changing legal status of marijuana across jurisdictions raises some valuable questions for marketing in sport, it also serves as a template for other drugs that may transition from being illicit to licit. For example, marijuana could be the drug that drives model policy for licit drug brand sports marketing activity aimed at preserving community interests in eliminating such marketing to children. Of course, doing so would likely require input from the range of stakeholders who take an interest in drug control-led integrity management in sport (see Chapters 5, 6 and 7).

Marketing licit drugs in sport

The marketing implications of drug control-led integrity management for sport are a potent mix of opportunities and risks. Sport stands to have mutually profitable ongoing relationships with licit drugs so long as it can sensitively and adaptively navigate the changing status of drugs. In doing so, sport needs to take responsibility for the effects those relationships have across the range of stakeholder interests. For example, sport does need to take responsibility for and be sensitive to the fact that it represents a key platform for marketing to children's and youth markets. Sport also needs to be very careful to ensure that it maintains a marketing portfolio across sin and non-sin products, or risk ceding control to dominant sponsors (Crompton, 2014). The insights derived from marketing licit drugs in sport potentially generalise to other sin products, such as gambling, both in terms of stakeholder interests and avoiding becoming dependent on sin-related revenue streams.

Drug scandals in sport

Scandal has become a regular phenomenon associated with sport. In terms of integrity management, scandal can arise when there is a violation of the rules- or values-based expectations that underpin the trust relationship between producers and consumers. This can happen for both individuals and institutions.

The Lance Armstrong case is perhaps one of the most prominent examples of a sports drug-related scandal impacting on an individual. During his career, Armstrong met the rules- and values-based expectations of sports producers and consumers through a carefully managed portrayal of the ideal qualities of a successful athlete. These qualities included a remarkable capacity to win high-profile events, overcoming testicular cancer and generous charity service, making Armstrong an ideal target for sponsorship. Despite denials to the contrary, Armstrong was eventually sanctioned for doping, violating the trust both producers and consumers had placed in him. As a consequence, Armstrong's value as a sports property evaporated.

The experiences of the IAAF represent an example of institutional drug-related scandal. As noted in Chapter 7, the German documentaries and subsequent Independent Commission (Pound, McLaren, & Younger, 2015) demonstrated the IAAF had violated the rules- and values-based expectations of producers and consumers. While doping was a catalyst for the scandal, the violation in the trust relationship appears to be one of systemic corruption of governance very similar to that reported in the Essendon Football Club (see Chapters 4 and 7). Both Adidas and Nestlé attributed their withdrawal from multi-year, multi-million dollar sponsorship of the IAAF to the doping scandal.

While both cases are powerful examples of drug-related scandal, the scandal construct has been notoriously difficult to define (Hughes & Shank, 2005). The components of a scandal are more apparent (see Prior *et al.*, 2013). First, the 'act' refers to the ways in which the actor violates rules- and/or values-based expectations. The impact of the act is likely to relate to its content, its frequency and how deliberate attempts were at concealment. If the act involves a severe violation, it is likely to generate a more profound reaction from sports consumers. For example, doping might have a harsher effect than being found to have misused sleeping pills. If the act occurs frequently, this is also likely to have a more profound effect over time unless deemed socially acceptable. For example, alcohol abuse commonly seen across the various versions of 'football' (e.g. soccer, union, league, grid iron or Australian Rules) rarely causes negative consumer reaction unless it is paired with another violation, such as violence or indecent behaviour. If the act was concealed and is discovered, the 'surprise effect' amplifies the reaction. For example, the concealment of doping for both Armstrong and the IAAF meant the surprise effect saw rapid magnification of the scandals.

A second major element of scandal is media attention. For most scandals, media coverage means the story can spread quickly and indiscriminately (e.g. to people who otherwise have no interest in sport). Given the increasing penetration and prominence of social media, a scandal can dominate social discourse within moments of its revelation (cf. Hambrick & Pegoraro, 2014). This then leads to conventional media such as television and newspapers picking up the story in pursuit of sensational content.

A third major element of scandal relates to corporate attempts to manage the scandal. In most cases, a sports organisation attempts to reduce the effects of the scandal. Since sports sponsors invest in a brand image, scandals usually alter this image considerably, often over a short period. This leads to the withdrawal of sponsorship. Indeed, sports sponsors often include contract clauses that allow them to withdraw quickly and with limited penalty in the wake of a scandal (Westberg, Stavros,

& Wilson, 2011). A scandal usually encourages most sponsors to withdraw immediately without facing contract termination penalties. Indeed, many sports sponsors adopt a standard approach to scandal management that involves (i) reducing the likelihood of scandal through athlete screening (although, see Chapter 9), (ii) minimising any damage through contract clauses and, (iii) instantly shifting their advertising and promotional approach in the wake of scandal.

In considering the broader marketing literature, scandal management could learn from other examples of customer promise violations such as product harm crises (Cleeren, Dekimpe, & Helsen, 2008; Cleeren, Van Heerde, & Dekimpe, 2013; Dawar & Pillutla, 2000) and service failures (Sajtos, Brodie, & Whittome, 2010; Gelbrich, 2010). In addition to other risk mitigation approaches, sports organisations are likely to survive scandals where sports consumers strongly identify with the athlete or sports entity. Sports fans have strong feelings of loyalty to a club or to individual athletes (Funk *et al.*, 2008), which is likely to buffer the effects of scandal. Another approach, similar to product recall, is for sponsors to instantly fire the player (e.g. Blumrodt & Ktichen, 2015). Successful product recalls involve attempts to address the fundamental problem before attempting a re-launch, which could also apply to drug-related scandal. Once a scandal has occurred, it is often an opportunity for the Chief Executive Officer of the sports organisation to lead the media through the scandal. A good approach is to admit the scandal and be explicit about its causes, followed by explanation of an action plan to address the causes, and finally offer a remediation approach which may involve compensating consumers in some way. Thus, an important part of the process is to address governance concerns that may arise from the scandal (see Chapter 7). The lessons from managing product harm crises and service failures also indicate that the aftermath of a scandal is the time to increase promotions and advertising activity.

While scandal management (including drug-related scandals) is difficult to manage, there is scope for the sports organisation to emerge better off than before. The scandal management process could provide an opportunity to eliminate difficult athletes from a roster. The increased marketing efforts are also means to re-establish connections with sports fans. As such, a scandal may be a blessing in disguise. As argued in Chapter 5, the management of a scandal can actually increase the share price of publically listed sports organisations (Mazanov, Lo Tenero, Connor, & Sharpe, 2012).

Managing drugs scandals

While violations of rules- or values-based expectations can have a negative impact on the value proposition of sports-related marketing arising from scandal, it can also have a positive impact. Indeed, the constantly evolving rules and values in relation to the role of drugs in sport and society make drug-related scandals, from licit drugs to doping, inevitable. As a result, sports managers need to plan for athlete and institutional drug-related scandals as part of their broader marketing and strategic planning (Connor & Mazanov, 2010). In doing so, there is significant scope for other sectors to learn about the marketing implications of scandal from sport.

Anti-doping as marketing

While it is easy to think of anti-doping in terms of its intended effects or management structures, anti-doping is also a powerful marketing device that communicates a set of principles and actions in relation to integrity, sport, drugs and performance enhancement. In terms of principles, anti-doping establishes a set of normative values that characterise what sport and society should consider to be virtuous (see Chapter 6), should consider to be sport (Jedlicka, 2014), should consider legitimate and illegitimate drugs (see Chapter 2), and should consider legitimate and illegitimate performance enhancement (see Chapter 1). In terms of actions, anti-doping establishes what sport and society should consider acceptable in pursuit of those normative values, ranging from administration of drug testing to public disclosures of sanctions to excluding athletes from decision making to censoring contradictory evidence and debate (cf. Møller, 2014). As a marketing device, anti-doping summarises the complexity of integrity management in sport, and in other contexts, acts as quality assurance of purity and goodness. That is, the presence of anti-doping assures producers and consumers that the integrity of sport has been protected.

Marketing to institutions

As argued in Chapter 7, the marketing of anti-doping has been extraordinarily successful at the systemic level, but has largely failed at the organisational and individual levels. It may be possible that anti-doping is an institutional rather than individual marketing device. That is, anti-doping was designed to market sports integrity to institutional stakeholders (e.g. sports federations, governments, broadcasters and sponsors) rather than individuals (e.g. athletes or fans). The enthusiasm for anti-doping at the institutional level is demonstrated by the volume of signatories to the relevant conventions and the World Anti-Doping Code (Houlihan, 2014). This may be because institutions derive value from an association with anti-doping in the same way licit drug manufacturers exploit halo effects from sport; association with anti-doping is to market the perception that a government or sport has addressed integrity issues in the most profound way possible. For example, the IAAF was a strong advocate for anti-doping (Wagner, 2011), presumably as part of a public relations plan to restore perceived integrity in the athletics brand following repeated doping scandals in the late twentieth century (which has some irony given the scandal of the early twenty-first century). The value of anti-doping for institutions also emerges from its absence (as argued in Chapter 1), where absence raises uncertainty about the rules- and values-based integrity of a sport. For example, discourses arising from the International Mixed Martial Arts Federation adoption of anti-doping focused on the sport transitioning towards a more certain future with regards to integrity. Institutions therefore stand to benefit from associating with anti-doping.

In comparison, individuals are unlikely to achieve much benefit from associating with anti-doping. For example, individual athletes are unlikely to benefit from associating themselves with anti-doping, because, no matter what they do, athletes are always under suspicion of doping (Kayser, 2011). The only time individual athletes may benefit from associating with anti-doping occurs immediately after an athlete has been sanctioned for doping. The association with anti-doping represents part of the public relations strategy to protect and rebuild the value of the athlete as a marketable sports property (see above). In terms of consumers, while stated preferences indicate firm convictions around the importance of drug control in sport (Engelberg, Moston, & Skinner, 2012; Solberg, Hanstad, & Thøring, 2010; Stamm, Lamprecht, Kamber, Marti, & Mahler, 2008), revealed preferences indicate doping has little impact on consumption patterns across attendance, broadcast (see Chapters 1 and 6) or even stock returns of sponsored products associated with a doping scandal (Danylchuk, Stegink, & Lebel, 2016). Given the apparently limited value of anti-doping to athletes and consumers, anti-doping may have more value when marketing to institutions rather than marketing to individuals.

Problems with a powerful marketing device

The power of anti-doping as a marketing device makes the management of integrity in sport easier in some regards, but also creates difficulties. One problem with the power of anti-doping draws on Levermore's (2013) observations around 'greenwashing' in sport. Greenwashing in this context means anti-doping being used in strategic communication to manage public perceptions by misleading or distracting stakeholders about integrity of sport issues. Anti-doping can be used to mislead producers and consumers that the integrity of sport is being protected despite evidence of widespread doping (see Chapter 8), as appears to have happened in the years prior to the revelations of widespread doping in international athletics. The marketing of anti-doping could also be used to distract stakeholders from other issues that relate to the integrity of sport. For example, the aggressive promotion of anti-doping has come at the expense of integrity issues arising from other types of drugs, and the expense of integrity issues such as governance failures, discrimination and exploitation (see Chapter 11). This raises the troubling implication that the symbolic value of anti-doping may exceed or has exceeded the practical value of implementing drug control for sport. Such an implication offers one explanation for the enthusiasm institutions show for adopting anti-doping at the expense of investing in anti-doping activity (see Chapter 7).

A second difficulty is that there may be more interest in protecting the integrity of anti-doping than in the integrity of sport. A core motivator for this is that anti-doping has value well beyond any individual sport or country, as a symbol of drug control-led integrity across sports and countries. For example, while revelations of widespread doping in athletics should have seen anti-doping critiqued for failing to implement meaningful drug control, the blame appears to have been placed upon corruption in the IAAF (Pound *et al.*, 2015). Protecting the value of anti-doping as a marketing device at the expense of the integrity of sport becomes unsettling when considering Møller's (2014) observations about corrupt idealism in the anti-doping movement, such that corrupt practices are seen as necessary evils in order to achieve the superordinate virtuous goal of doping-free sport. For example, the IAAF and WADA suppression of a report which indicated widespread doping across international athletics championships (BBC, 2015) suggests a willingness to protect anti-doping rather than protect the integrity of sport. Part of the reason for this is that anything which threatens anti-doping threatens the integrity of all the institutions associated with anti-doping. On this logic, it makes sense to place the blame on the IAAF, as it means the integrity of anti-doping remains viable for other signatories. Of course, this sort of behaviour contradicts the principles of CSR that underpin integrity management in the first place.

A third problem with making anti-doping such a powerful marketing device is to consider the implications should sport move to a different drug control policy (see Chapter 12). For example, the anti-doping policy has prompted increasing interest in what constitutes integrity in sport (see Chapter 6), one outcome of which may be that drug control-led integrity management is unnecessary. Alternatively, changing social norms around the role of drugs in society may force sport to redevelop its understanding of the role drugs play in both sport and the integrity of sport. The prospect of having to invest resources into changing marketing activity away from anti-doping may create institutional inertia and therefore a reluctance to change. Like the drug crises that presaged anti-doping in the first place (see Chapter 3), it may take another series of crises to compel sport to overcome the power of anti-doping as a high-value marketing device.

Managing the marketing of anti-doping

The growing strength of anti-doping as a symbol of integrity management is a double-edged sword. One edge means that countries and institutions clamour to be associated with anti-doping, further increasing its strength and influence. The other edge means that anti-doping needs to be carefully managed to maintain its value as a marketing device. Like any marketing activity, the marketing proposition offered by anti-doping stands to be misappropriated or exploited in ways that potentially undermine its value as a symbol of integrity management, even when those actions are intended to promote integrity in sport. This creates the risk that any diminution in anti-doping leads to a diminution of integrity in sport. As a consequence, the value of anti-doping as a marketing device also needs to be managed with the same level of integrity that anti-doping seeks to achieve through drug control-led integrity management.

Marketing drugs and integrity in sport

Marketing clearly has a key role to play in drug control-led integrity in sport, which makes its omission from texts on sports marketing all the more surprising. The experiences sport has had engaging in marketing relationships with sin products offer potent lessons for other market sectors, both in terms of being aware of and meeting the responsibility to other stakeholders, and avoiding being over-reliant on a single marketing revenue stream. Management of drug scandal in sport should form part of both strategic and operational planning for both institutions and individual sports properties. In doing so, the experience of managing such scandal offers a rich skein of data to inform the implications of scandal on integrity management across market sectors. Finally, drug control-led integrity management has imbued anti-doping with significant power as a marketing device. In doing so, sport needs to be very careful about how that marketing device is managed. A difficult challenge lies in determining how to manage the protection of anti-doping relative to protecting the integrity of sport, which remains a challenge for any integrity-related organisation (e.g. Transparency International). This represents a valuable cross-over point where integrity practice in sport can both inform and learn from integrity efforts in other market sectors.

References

BBC (2015). IAAF accused of suppressing athletes' doping study. Available at: www.bbc.co.uk/sport/athletics/33948924 (accessed 7 Feb 2016).

Belt, O., Stamatakos, K., Ayers, A. J., Fryer, V. A., Jernigan, D. H., & Siegel, M. (2014). Vested interests in addiction research and policy. Alcohol brand sponsorship of events, organizations and causes in the United States, 2010–2013. *Addiction*, *109*(12), 1977–1985.

Blumrodt, J., & Kitchen, P. J. (2015). The Tour de France: Corporate sponsorships and doping accusations. *Journal of Business Strategy, 36*(2), 41–48.

Chadwick, S., Chanavat, N., & Desbordes, M. (Eds.). (2016). *Routledge Handbook of Sports Marketing*. Abingdon: Routledge.

Cleeren, K., Dekimpe, M. G., & Helsen, K. (2008). Weathering product-harm crises. *Journal of the Academy of Marketing Science, 36*(2), 262–270.

Cleeren, K., Van Heerde, H. J., & Dekimpe, M. G. (2013). Rising from the ashes: How brands and categories can overcome product-harm crises. *Journal of Marketing, 77*(2), 58–77.

Coleman, B., Johnson, S., Tessman, G., Tworek, C., Alexander, J., Dickinson, D., *et al.* (2016). 'It's not smoke. It's not tar. It's not 4000 chemicals. Case closed': Exploring attitudes, beliefs, and perceived social norms of e-cigarette use among adult users. *Drug and Alcohol Dependence, 159*(1), 80–85.

Connor, J. M., & Mazanov, J. (2010). The inevitability of scandal: Lessons for sponsors and administrators. *International Journal of Sports Marketing and Sponsorship, 11*(3), 29–37.

Crompton, J. L. (2014). Potential negative outcomes from sponsorship for a sport property. *Managing Leisure, 19*(6), 420–441.

Danylchuk, K., Stegink, J., & Lebel, K. (2016). Doping scandals in professional cycling: Impact on primary team sponsor's stock return. *International Journal of Sports Marketing and Sponsorship, 17*(1), 37–55.

Davidson, D. K. (2003). *Selling Sin: The Marketing of Socially Unacceptable Products*. Westport, CT: Greenwood Publishing.

Dawar, N., & Pillutla, M. M. (2000). Impact of product-harm crises on brand equity: The moderating role of consumer expectations. *Journal of Marketing Research, 37*(2), 215–226.

Dawes, J. (2014). Cigarette brand loyalty and purchase patterns: An examination using US consumer panel data. *Journal of Business Research, 67*(9), 1933–1943.

De Andrade, M., Hastings, G., Angus, K., Dixon, D., & Purves, R. (2013). *The Marketing of Electronic Cigarettes in the UK*. Available at: https://dspace.stir.ac.uk/bitstream/1893/17889/1/deAndradeetale-cigsreport.pdf (accessed 4 February 2016).

Del Coso, J., Lara, B., & López-Muñoz, F. (2015). Caffeinated energy drinks boost physical performance in several sport modalities: Should they be considered by anti-doping authorities? *Clinical and Experimental Pharmacology, 5*(2).

Duchan, E., Patel, N. D., & Feucht, C. (2010). Energy drinks: A review of use and safety for athletes. *The Physician and Sportsmedicine, 38*(2), 171–179.

Emond, J. A., Sargent, J. D., & Gilbert-Diamond, D. (2015). Patterns of energy drink advertising over US television networks. *Journal of Nutrition Education and Behavior, 47*(2), 120–126.

Engelberg, T., Moston, S., & Skinner, J. (2012). Public perception of sport anti-doping policy in Australia. *Drugs: Education, Prevention and Policy, 19*(1), 84–87.

Fairchild, A. L., Bayer, R., & Colgrove, J. (2014). The renormalization of smoking? E-cigarettes and the tobacco 'endgame'. *New England Journal of Medicine, 370*(4), 293–295.

Fischer, B., Kuganesan, S., & Room, R. (2015). Medical Marijuana programs: Implications for cannabis control policy–Observations from Canada. *International Journal of Drug Policy, 26*(1), 15–19.

Funk, D., Alexandris, K., & McDonald, H. (2008). *Consumer Behaviour in Sport and Events*. Abingdon: Routledge.

Gelbrich, K. (2010). Anger, frustration, and helplessness after service failure: Coping strategies and effective informational support. *Journal of the Academy of Marketing Science, 38*(5), 567–585.

Hambrick, M. E., & Pegoraro, A. (2014). Social Sochi: Using social network analysis to investigate electronic word-of-mouth transmitted through social media communities. *International Journal of Sport Management and Marketing, 15*(3–4), 120–140.

Hanstad, D. V., & Waddington, I. (2009). Sport, health and drugs: A critical re-examination of some key issues and problems. *Perspectives in Public Health, 129*(4), 174–182.

Harris, J. L., & Munsell, C. R. (2015). Energy drinks and adolescents: What's the harm? *Nutrition Reviews, 73*(4), 247–257.

Houlihan, B. (2014). Achieving compliance in international anti-doping policy: An analysis of the 2009 World Anti-Doping Code. *Sport Management Review, 17*(3), 265–276.

Hughes, S., & Shank, M. (2005). Defining scandal in sports: Media and corporate sponsor perspectives. *Sport Marketing Quarterly, 14*(4), 207–216.

Jedlicka, S. (2014). The normative discourse of anti-doping policy. *International Journal of Sport Policy and Politics, 6*(3), 429–442.

Jones, S. C. (2010). When does alcohol sponsorship of sport become sports sponsorship of alcohol? A case study of developments in sport in Australia. *International Journal of Sports Marketing and Sponsorship, 11*(3), 67–78.

Kalkhoran, S., & Glantz, S. A. (2016). E-cigarettes and smoking cessation in real world settings: A systematic review and meta-analysis. *The Lancet Respiratory Medicine, 4*(2), 116–128.

Kayser, B. (2011). On the presumption of guilt without proof and intentionality and other consequences of current anti-doping policy. In M. McNamee & V. Møller (Eds.), *Doping and Anti-Doping Policy in Sport: Ethical, Legal and Social Perspectives* (pp. 84–99). Abingdon: Routledge.

Kornfield, R., Huang, J., Vera, L., & Emery, S. L. (2015). Rapidly increasing promotional expenditures for e-cigarettes. *Tobacco Control, 24*(2), 110–111.

Lamont, M., Hing, N., & Gainsbury, S. (2011). Gambling on sport sponsorship: A conceptual framework for research and regulatory review. *Sport Management Review, 14*(3), 246–257.

Levermore, R. (2013). Viewing CSR through sport from a critical perspective: Failing to address gross corporate misconduct? In J. Paramio-Salcines, K. Babiak, & G. Walters (Eds.), *Routledge Handbook of Sport and Corporate Social Responsibility* (pp. 52–61). Abingdon: Routledge.

Lindsay, S., Thomas, S., Lewis, S., Westberg, K., Moodie, R., & Jones, S. (2013). Eat, drink and gamble: Marketing messages about 'risky' products in an Australian major sporting series. *BMC Public Health, 13*(1), 1.

Mallen, C., & Mansurov, A. (2015). Sport sponsorship and the Canadian medical marijuana industry. *Journal of Sports Management and Commercialization, 5*(2), 1–12.

Mazanov, J., Huybers, T., & Connor, J. (2012). Prioritising health in anti-doping: What Australians think. *Journal of Science and Medicine in Sport, 15*(5), 381–385.

Mazanov, J., Lo Tenero, G., Connor, J., & Sharpe, K. (2012). Scandal + football = a better share price. *Sport, Business and Management*, 2(2), 92–114.

McDaniel, S., Mason, D., & Kinney, L. (2004). Spectator sport's strange bedfellows: The commercial sponsorship of sporting events to promote tobacco, alcohol and lotteries. In T. Stack (Ed.), *The Commercialisation of Sport* (pp. 287–305). Abingdon: Routledge.

McGhee, T. (2012). The rise and rise of athlete brand endorsements. *Journal of Brand Strategy*, 1(1), 79–84.

McKee, M. (2013). E-cigarettes and the marketing push that surprised everyone. *British Medical Journal*, 2013, 347: f5780.

Meier, P. S. (2011). Alcohol marketing research: The need for a new agenda. *Addiction*, 106(3), 466–471.

Møller, V. (2014). Who guards the guardians? *International Journal of the History of Sport*, 31(8), 934–950.

Pepper, J. K., Emery, S. L., Ribisl, K. M., Rini, C. M., & Brewer, N. T. (2015). How risky is it to use e-cigarettes? Smokers' beliefs about their health risks from using novel and traditional tobacco products. *Journal of Behavioral Medicine*, 38(2), 318–326.

Pomeranz, J. L., Munsell, C. R., & Harris, J. L. (2013). Energy drinks: an emerging public health hazard for youth. *Journal of Public Health Policy*, 34(2), 254–271.

Pound, R., McLaren, R., & Younger, G. (2015). *Independent Commission Report #1*. Montreal: World Anti-Doping Agency.

Prior, D., O'Reilly, N., Mazanov, J., & Huybers, T. (2013). The impact of scandal on sport consumption: a conceptual framework for future research. *International Journal of Sport Management and Marketing*, 14(1–4), 188–211.

Reissig, C. J., Strain, E. C., & Griffiths, R. R. (2009). Caffeinated energy drinks – a growing problem. *Drug and Alcohol Dependence*, 99(1), 1–10.

Reszel, R. (2011). Guilty until proven innocent, and then, still guilty: What the World Anti-Doping Agency can learn from the National Football League about first-time anti-doping violations. *Wisconsin International Law Journal*, 29(4), 807–832.

Sajtos, L., Brodie, R. J., & Whittome, J. (2010). Impact of service failure: The protective layer of customer relationships. *Journal of Service Research*, 13(2), 216–229.

Sanchis-Gomar, F., Pareja-Galeano, H., Cervellin, G., Lippi, G., & Earnest, C. P. (2015). Energy drink overconsumption in adolescents: Implications for arrhythmias and other cardiovascular events. *Canadian Journal of Cardiology*, 31(57), 2e575.

Siegel, M., Chen, K., DeJong, W., Naimi, T. S., Ostroff, J., Ross, C. S., et al. (2015). Differences in alcohol brand consumption between underage youth and adults – United States, 2012. *Substance Abuse*, 36(1), 106–112.

Solberg, H. A., Hanstad, D. V., & Thøring, T. A. (2010). Doping in elite sport – do the fans care? Public opinion on the consequences of doping scandals. *International Journal of Sports Marketing and Sponsorship*, 11(3), 2–16.

Stamm, H., Lamprecht, M., Kamber, M., Marti, B., & Mahler, N. (2008). The public perception of doping in sport in Switzerland, 1995–2004. *Journal of Sports Sciences*, 26(3), 235–242.

Thorpe, H. (2012). 'Sex, drugs and snowboarding': (Il)legitimate definitions of taste and lifestyle in a physical youth culture. *Leisure Studies*, *31*(1), 33–51.

Trumbo, C. W., & Harper, R. (2015). Orientation of US young adults toward e-cigarettes and their use in public. *Health Behavior and Policy Review*, *2*(2), 163–170.

Wagner, U. (2011). Towards the construction of the world anti-doping agency: Analyzing the approaches of FIFA and the IAAF to doping in sport. *European Sport Management Quarterly*, *11*(5), 445–470.

Wang, R. T., & Kaplanidou, K. (2013). I want to buy more because I feel good: The effect of sport-induced emotion on sponsorship. *International Journal of Sports Marketing and Sponsorship*, *15*(1), 52–66.

Westberg, K., Stavros, C., & Wilson, B. (2011). The impact of degenerative episodes on the sponsorship B2B relationship: Implications for brand management. *Industrial Marketing Management*, *40*(4), 603–611.

Part III

Drug control-led integrity management

Chapter 11

Managing drugs beyond elite male sport

Like many other aspects of sport, the discussion and evidence around managing drugs in sport tends to default to elite male sport. For example, Aubel and Ohl's (2014) discussion of how doping is managed in cycling did so from the perspective of male professional cycling. This has seen discussion and evidence about the management of drugs for other versions of sport ignored. Ignoring other versions of sport may violate the obligations imposed by the pursuit of corporate social responsibility (CSR) in sport (see Chapter 1), and therefore undermine the ability to manage integrity in sport. The management of drugs in three other versions of sport is therefore considered: women's sport, children's sport and non-elite sport. The consideration of other versions of sport suggests that drug control-led integrity management for sport may need to specifically account for variation in how drugs and drug control are experienced across women's, children's and non-elite sport.

Managing drugs in women's sport

Sport is well known for reinforcing the gender hierarchy, such that male sport is treated as the standard by which women's sport is judged inferior (Lenskyj, 2003; Pfister, 2010; Schneider, 2010). This is replicated across sport, from male-dominated boards to lower pay for female athletes to unnecessarily sexualising female athlete uniforms (e.g. Flake, Durfur, & Moore, 2013; Kenny & Bell, 2011; Magdalinski, 2009). While empirical studies which establish that the gender hierarchy repeats for sports drug control are yet to be conducted, the indications are that the gender hierarchy is repeated. This argument is advanced by presenting evidence that men and women use drugs for sport differently. The argument then examines how the gender neutral approach to drug control offered by the World Anti-Doping Code (the Code) violates the principle of policy harmonisation by treating women differently. The argument concludes by observing that women's experience of drug control in sport appears to support theorising about gender in organisations, and compromises the integrity of women's sport.

Women's use of drugs for sport

Gender remains one of the most consistent predictors of drug use, misuse and abuse. In simple terms, males and females consistently demonstrate different patterns of drug consumption. For example, males and females display very different patterns of smoking tobacco, with more men smoking than women (Ng *et al.*, 2014). Gender differences in prevalence, patterns of use and reasons for use appear similar across combustible and e-cigarettes (Piñeiro *et al.*, 2016). Differences also emerge for caffeine (men consume, on average, more than women; Penolazzi, Natale, Leone, & Russo, 2012) and alcohol (although gender gaps appear to be narrowing; Dawson, Goldstein, Saha, & Grant, 2015; Keyes, Li, & Hasin, 2011). The evidence indicates women are more likely to misuse prescription drugs (Boyd *et al.*, 2015; Simoni-Wastila, 2000), although men are more likely to die as a result of overdose (Paulozzi, Jones, Mack, & Rudd, 2011). Women use fewer illicit drugs, and are less likely to engage in poly drug use (e.g. combining prescription drugs with illicit drug use; Kelly, Wells, Pawson, LeClair, & Parsons, 2014). Men are more likely to die from an overdose of illicit drugs (Paulozzi *et al.*, 2011).

Athlete populations show slightly different patterns of drug use. Sports participation correlates with lower use across most drugs, with the exceptions being alcohol (athletes tend to drink more dangerously than the general population; Green, Nelson, & Hartmann, 2014; Kwan, Bobko, Faulkner, Donnelly, & Cairney, 2014), supplements and doping (Yusko, Buckman, White, & Pandina, 2008). Drug use for sport also varies significantly across genders, with the prevalence rates of using supplements and illicit drugs higher among male athletes (Dunn, Thomas, Swift, & Burns, 2011; Schaal *et al.*, 2011). Women tend to use supplements for aesthetic (e.g. weight control) or health reasons rather than performance enhancement (Jordan & Naclerio, 2014; Mazanov, Petróczi, Bingham, & Holloway, 2008; Weaving & Teetzel, 2014). The exception appears to be prescription drugs, with female athletes reporting greater rates of use than male athletes (Suzic *et al.* 2011). In terms of doping, noting that drug testing by anti-doping agencies is widely regarded as underestimating doping prevalence, the 2013 Anti-Doping Rule Violations Report produced by WADA shows that 330 of the 1,687 adverse analytical findings (detection of a prohibited substance in a sample) came from females, suggesting men dope at five times the rate of women. (It is impossible to ascertain how many of the 207,513 tested samples came from men and women). This is consistent with self-report evidence which shows males more likely to dope than females (Papadopoulos, Skalkidis, Parkkari, & Petridou, 2006). Moreover, evidence indicates that men and women have fundamentally different patterns of doping across career trajectories (Pitsch & Emrich, 2012).

These results indicate that the patterns of drug use among women in sports contexts are different to the way men use drugs for sport. Indeed, the difference in usage patterns suggests that universal drug control would more properly address alcohol misuse and abuse. Beyond alcohol, men's sport should invest in control for performance enhancing supplements, illicit drugs and doping, which is the main focus for anti-doping. Drug control for women's sport would more usefully address supplement use for health enhancement and the role of prescription drugs in sport.

Gender and the Code

Despite the apparent gender differences in drug use generally and doping specifically, the Code is silent on the issue of gender. Indeed, none of the words 'male', 'female' or 'gender' appear in the Code. Taken at face value, this is consistent with policy harmonisation such that anti-doping should be experienced the same way irrespective of gender. However, brief consideration of drug testing, out-of-competition testing and the implications of sanctions demonstrates women have a fundamentally different experience of drug control in sport to men.

Drug testing requires athletes to be naked from nipple to knee, and a person with delegated authority has to witness the sample leaving the urethra and entering the sample collection vessel. While there is no question the sample collection process can be a confronting and degrading experience for both genders (e.g. Henne, 2015), half of women find the experience distressing compared to one third of men (Efverström, Ahmadi, Bavkström, & Hoff, 2014). That is, women are disproportionately affected by drug testing. It remains to be seen whether the approach taken to drug testing would be sustained if half of all men tested found the experience degrading and distressing.

The approach to drug testing taken by anti-doping raises the spectre of gender testing. Gender testing was introduced to protect the integrity of sport from men posing as women, including infamous parades where female athletes were forced to line up to have their genitalia medically scrutinised (Cooky, Dycus, & Dworkin, 2013; Henne, 2015). This approach was eventually repealed on the basis that it was degrading and inequitable to women (Heggie, 2010; Karkazis, Jordan-Young, Davis, & Camporesi, 2012). Given the parallels between gender testing and drug testing, the argument that the method of drug testing employed under the Code is disproportionately degrading and inequitable to women is both plausible and potentially powerful.

The implications of out-of-competition testing could also disproportionately affect women. Out-of-competition testing means athletes must nominate, three months in advance, one hour of every day (some countries restrict the hours, others require 24-hour availability), a place they will be available for an unannounced drug test. Athletes who are unavailable at the nominated time and place can be sanctioned. The restrictions on freedom of movement imposed by out-of-competition testing mean athletes who may be required to be elsewhere at short notice may be compromised. For example, athletes involved in volunteer firefighting risk being sanctioned for defending a property from fire when they should be available for out-of-competition testing. The gendered nature of this principle emerges when considering women bear the majority of the burden for child rearing. While the combination of an athletic career and motherhood has been traditionally discouraged (Palmer & Leberman, 2009), the number of women who combine a career as an elite athlete with motherhood is growing (McGannon, Gonsalves, Schinke, & Busanich, 2015). This could see a mother sanctioned as unavailable for out-of-competition testing while responding to a request to pick up their sick child from school. This suggests that out-of-competition testing could lead to unequal treatment of the genders.

Should an athlete face sanctions under the Code, it has been argued that the relatively shorter career of female athletes means a sanction for doping is more likely to end their careers (e.g. Amos & Fridman, 2009). At the time of writing, research on career length in individual professional sport was still emerging (Frick, Humphreys, & Scheel, 2015, p. 152), with remarkably little data on women's sporting careers (comparative or otherwise). The absence of direct data compels inferring the gendered impact of a sanction from indirect data. Evidence suggests that European male athletic careers are, on average, 2.7 years longer than female careers (Stambulova, Stephan, & Jäphag, 2007). Assuming the same holds true for professional basketball in the United States, the average eight-year career for men (Baker, Koz, Kungl, Fraser-Thomas, & Schorer, 2013) becomes a five-year career for women. This suggests that, although significantly disrupted, a male basketball player's career can survive a doping ban, whereas a doping ban would see a female career end. Standardised sanctions therefore appear to impact the sporting careers of women in a different way to men's careers.

Gender neutrality and drug control

These three examples suggest that, rather than ensuring drug control is experienced the same by everyone (equality), the Code creates some significant inequities on the basis of gender. Theorising around the role of gender in organisations describes the Code's silence on gender concealing inequities as 'gender neutrality' in policy (Korvajarvi, 2011). The absence of gender from a policy is meant to imply neutrality in the sense that all those affected by the policy are treated equally under the policy. In doing so, silence on gender means the policy conceals the gender hierarchy with the consequence that the hierarchy is reproduced and women's interest systematically compromised. It seems that the pursuit of policy harmonisation has led to unintended gender neutrality. This indicates that drug control for sport needs to address how it promotes the integrity of women and women's sport as part of the process.

A different approach is for women's sport to develop an alternative approach to drug control. This approach, drawn from the radical feminist literature, argues that, given sport is already segregated by gender, women can develop their own independent version of sport (Lenskyj, 2003). In terms of drug control, this would mean developing a system aimed at the drugs most likely to be misused or abused by female athletes (e.g. prescription drugs), using urinary dye markers instead of distressing witnessed drug tests (see Elbe *et al.*, 2016), and sanctions commensurate to the female sporting career.

Managing drugs in children's sport

Experimentation with drugs is a feature of adolescence, and has been the focus of intensive research and practice to prevent, delay onset or educate adolescents about drug use. For some substances (e.g. alcohol, supplements, over-the-counter drugs and prescription drugs), interventions are aimed at promoting use and managing misuse while preventing abuse. For other substances (e.g. tobacco, illicit drugs and doping), interventions are predicated on abstinence given profound public health and societal consequences (e.g. China's eighteenth and nineteenth century opium crisis). These interventions are complemented by policies aimed at controlling supply (e.g. making it illegal to sell cigarettes to minors) or demand (e.g. anti-doping sanctions). Despite the combinations of interventions and policies to manage adolescent drug consumption, the majority of drug behaviour still has its roots in adolescence. Sport is no different; the genesis of drug use in sport has its roots in adolescence.

Normalising and use of drugs in children's and adolescent sport

It is important to remember that all children and adolescents have to navigate the role drugs play in their lives. For the most part, as noted above, sports participation is correlated with lower rates of use across most drugs, with an apparent aversion to smoking and illicit drug use due to their performance diminishing effects (Lisha & Sussman, 2010).

Alcohol is a special case for sport given its role in socialising athletes into the hypermasculine ideals of sport. Stewart and Smith (2008) characterise the correlation between hypermasculinity and drugs in sport relative to Whitehead's (2005) heroism concept, which values both aggression and risk taking. The socialising process sees young athletes habituated to the ubiquitous presence of alcohol in sport, the dependence of sport on alcohol sponsorship and the role alcohol plays in social interactions for sport (e.g. consuming alcohol after an event). Alcohol misuse and abuse is reconstructed as a demonstration of hypermasculinity through 'heroic' binge drinking that requires aggressive and potentially damaging levels of consumption. The capacity of athletes to perform at peak levels following such binge drinking is also reconstructed as 'heroic' action. Given males can typically consume more alcohol than females, this activity also serves to reinforce the gender hierarchy.

When it comes to drugs that have specific sports-related implications, evidence from France (Lentillon-Kaestnar, & Carstairs, 2010; Lentillon-Kaestnar, Hagger, & Hardcastle, 2012) and Australia (Mazanov, Hemphill, Connor, Quirk, & Backhouse, 2015) indicates pre-adolescent children learn about the role of these drugs from the time they begin participating in sport. Child athletes and their parents are subjected to two narratives aimed at promoting drug use in sport. The first is aimed at socialising children and parents to use drugs when faced with illness or injury as part of the medicalisation of society. The second is socialising children and their parents that they need specialised drugs to medicate their participation in sport. This process parallels the medicalisation of society with the scientisation of sport, normalising the role and consumption of sports science. The focus for children's sport is normalising drug use for health rather than performance. For example, a medical practitioner may recommend supplements or prescribe drugs to manage fatigue arising from over training.

The evidence from French cycling (Ohl, Fincouer, Lentillon-Kaestnar, Defrance, & Brissonneau, 2015) suggests adolescent athletes transitioning to adult competition sees the introduction of drug use for performance. Supplement manufacturers exploit the expanding interest in performance enhancing drug use among junior athletes and their parents (and everyone else), marketing a range of products as performance enhancing without evidence to support those claims (see Chapter 5). It is open to debate whether performance enhancing supplements represent 'gateway' drugs that are a precursor to doping, but the evidence suggests that those who dope are also more likely to use supplements believed to be performance enhancing (Backhouse, Whitaker, & Petróczi, 2013; Hildebrandt, Harty, & Langenbucher, 2012; Papadopoulos et al., 2006; Petróczi, Mazanov, & Naughton, 2011).

It appears that doping is relatively rare in children's sport. Noting that drug test results are likely to underestimate true doping prevalence, the benchmark used to discuss doping in children's sport is the 2013 WADA analytical positive rate of 0.8 per cent. At the 2010 Singapore Summer Youth Olympic Games, two wrestlers were disqualified for using a prohibited diuretic (which is used to mask doping rather than being performance enhancing) out of the 1,231 tests conducted (IOC, 2010), indicating a 0.2 per cent detection rate. The 2014 Nanjing Summer Youth Olympic Games saw only one athlete tested positive for a diuretic out of 596 tests (again, 0.2 per cent) (IOC, 2014). The Summer Youth Olympic results correspond with those from Texan high school American Football. A moral panic about doping in high school football led to a sports drug control programme six times larger than drug testing for the 2008 Beijing Summer Olympic Games (Woolf & Swain, 2014). A total of 53,818 tests were conducted with only 22 confirmed positives (0.04 per cent, or one twentieth of the adult rate) and 154 unresolved cases or protocol violations (0.3 per cent). By comparison, there were no doping violations at either the Innsbruck (2012) or Lillehammer (2016) Winter Youth Olympic Games. At two successive Winter Youth Olympic Games doping was absent (or at least undetected or unprosecuted). The results across four Youth Olympics and a significant drug testing programme among Texan adolescents suggest that analytically confirmed doping is rarer among children than it is among adults.

These results indicate that drug control for children's sport would more usefully address the culture around alcohol misuse and abuse in the first instance, followed by a closer examination of the role of and culture around medicating the health effects of sports participation. Adolescent sport would benefit from greater investment in controlling supplements through both regulation of the supplement industry (e.g. evidence-based claims) and education about the role of supplements in sport (e.g. how to use caffeine safely).

Children and the Code

As with gender, the Code's adherence to the principles of policy harmonisation creates inequities for children involved in sport, and their parents. The arguments presented are based on reports that a nine-year-old was selected for drug testing in the United Kingdom (Hubbard, 2015). The Court of Arbitration for Sport (2006) is clear that 'it is not the age, sex or any other personal characteristics of an individual that determines the application of the anti-doping rules but the participation of an athlete in events governed by the rule'. As a result, it is appropriate to consider inequities as they arise to children of all ages. Three related inequities arising from the Code for children are addressed; consent, the impact of drug testing and the consequences of being sanctioned.

Two conditions to participation in the Youth Olympic Games provide a starting point for the discussion around consent; that athletes must be at least 15 years old to participate and that they are Code compliant (IOC, 2012). Given that the entire anti-doping architecture is predicated upon a system of agreements to be Code compliant, consent indicates understanding what Code compliance means. Understanding Code compliance can be thought of as being able to comprehend the role of drugs in sport, why doping is contrary to sports practice, the Prohibited List, what a drug test is and the consequences of an ADRV. For example, consent implies that children and their parents understand the implications of out-of-competition testing (e.g. a 6 a.m. unannounced drug test) and that they may be unable to access some therapeutic drugs as a result of their Code compliant status.

In the absence of direct assessment of adolescent athlete knowledge of the Code comparable with direct assessment of adults (e.g. Mazanov, Backhouse, Connor, Hemphill, & Quirk, 2014), the evidence from self-assessed level of knowledge suggests that adolescent athletes have, at best, a moderate level of understanding of the Code (Fürhapter *et al.*, 2013). Like adults with little knowledge of the Code, adolescent athletes tend to substitute a range of beliefs about the Code and the role of drugs in sport. For example, Code compliant young elite athletes in the United Kingdom (16–21 years old) tended to follow 'drugs are bad' tropes (e.g. Bloodworth & McNamee, 2010). Notably, at the time of writing, there was no evidence available on pre-adolescent athlete knowledge of the Code, and whether they have any understanding of what Code compliance means in terms of consent. However, the contractual basis of Code compliance means that children are unable to consent on their own behalf, which means that parental or guardian consent is used as a substitute. Unfortunately, parents and guardians were the least knowledgeable about the Code in a study of athlete support personnel (Mazanov *et al.*, 2014).

Neither children nor their parents or guardians appear to have sufficient insight into the Code to comprehend the implications of being compliant. This is particularly problematic when parents sign membership agreements or contracts on behalf of children engaging in junior participation sports. While most athletes who take part in junior participation sport never have any contact with anti-doping, it is unclear what role the implications of Code compliance play when parents sign professional playing contracts on behalf of children aged 18 months old, as has happened in Association Football (soccer) (BBC, 2011). As a consequence, both policy harmonisation and case law mean children holding a professional contract for sport can be treated just like any other professional athlete.

While there is evidence drug testing can be a distressing experience for adults, there is no evidence about how children respond to drug testing. Like an adult, a nine-year-old child is required to be naked from nipple to knee and have someone witness the sample leaving the urethra and entering the sample collection vessel. The child may become distressed and unable to produce a sample (known as paruresis) or may simply refuse to produce the sample. If a parent or guardian is present, they may be able to make the judgement that the harms associated with being sanctioned for an ADRV are lower than the distress of drug testing. However, a child who is away from their parents or guardians may be unable to make that judgement. In this instance, it would be hoped that the adult with a duty of care to the child, such as a coach or sports trainer, would act in the best interests of the child. Unfortunately, there is a potential conflict of interest given the coach or sports trainer has an obligation to protect and promote the Code. The child could legitimately object saying they never agreed to be part of drug control, which is irrelevant given their parent or guardian agreed on their behalf. While this set of circumstances may seem far-fetched, they happened to a 17-year-old female non-elite athlete in Germany, who ended up agreeing to be sanctioned rather than complete a drug test (Elbe, Schlegel, & Brand, 2012).

The third possible inequity relates to the consequences of being sanctioned. There is some evidence to suggest that being sanctioned under the Code causes some negative psychological reactions among athletes, including depression (Elbe & Overbye, 2015). There is no evidence as to children's psychological responses to being sanctioned. It is also unclear how sanctioning a child for violating the Code may impact their social health. For example, the association with an ADRV (Article 2.10) may preclude the child from playing sport with their friends, leading to social isolation and potentially stigmatisation among their friendship group. It is also unclear whether being sanctioned for an ADRV as a child has any implications for later life. For example, if it becomes known that a child was sanctioned, as was the case for the two young athletes who tested positive at the 2010 Youth Olympic Games, it may have an impact on their ability to get a job as an adult. While Article 14.3.6 provides an exemption for mandatory public disclosures in cases involving a child in the 2015 Code, it also prescribes that the exemption is subject to the facts and circumstances of the case. That is, the decision can be taken that sanctions for a minor can be made public if it is deemed to be in the interest of promoting the anti-doping ideology.

The way the Code treats children also has implications for parents and guardians. Parents and guardians have to be careful about the drugs they give their child. For example, a Tae Kwon Do trainer from Canada was sanctioned for inadvertently giving a junior athlete a prohibited over-the-counter drug (Canadian Centre for Ethics in Sport, 2012). It is easy to see how a parent or guardian could do something similar. Given the range of drugs governed by the Code, a parent or guardian giving their child a protein supplement contaminated with a diuretic may be sanctioned for supplying a prohibited drug (Article 2.8). Article 10.3.3 indicates that violations of Article 2.8 are particularly serious and compel a lifetime ban. Given Article 2.10 prevents other athletes and support personnel from associating with those sanctioned for the purposes of sport, the parent or guardian would no longer be able to be associated with the child's preparation for events or their sport (e.g. volunteering at events). Banning guardians from sport effectively bans the entire family.

Drug control in children's sport

The gender neutrality of the Code appears to extend to children's sport. It is clear that the role of drugs in children's sport is fundamentally different to the role of drugs in elite male sport. Designing drug control around elite male sport leads to inequitable outcomes for both children and their parents or guardians. Indeed, some have asked whether the inequitable treatment of children under the Code violates the basic rights of the child (Teetzel & Mazzucco, 2014). The failure to address how children engage with drugs in sport and the inequitable outcomes for children seems incongruous with claims that drug control contributes to the integrity of sport.

Managing drugs in non-elite sport

Non-elite sport encompasses the broad range of sports events that fall outside the resources of elite or professional sport, ranging from recreational sport through to organised events such as Masters Games. While elite or professional athletes may participate in such events (e.g. the World University Games), the majority of participants are amateurs for whom sport represents one of many careers (e.g. work, family and study) rather than the dominant career. Given the sheer volume of participants and breadth of events, implementing drug control for non-elite sport is a particular challenge. The anti-doping movement has attempted to reconstruct its private interest concerns around doping into a public health concern. In doing so, discussion about translating anti-doping from elite sport to all sport has made it clear that anti-doping is unfeasible as a form of drug control beyond the well-resourced elite.

Drugs in sport and society

While non-elite athletes may take an interest in sports specific drugs, it occurs alongside other drug careers. This includes functional drug use to manage work–life balance (e.g. parents using methylphenidate), to enable workplace activity (e.g. anabolic steroids use among police officers; Hoberman, 2005), socialising (e.g. alcohol or ecstasy) or medicinal use (e.g. marijuana for pain management). At the same time that sport has been trying to regain control over drugs there has been a steady increase in the number of illicit drug users (United Nations Office on Drugs and Crime, 2015) and alcohol consumption (World Health Organisation, 2014). Of interest to sport is the stabilisation of caffeine consumption (at least in the United

States; Fulgoni, Keast, & Lieberman, 2015) and decrease in the global use of anabolic-androgenic steroids (Sagoe, Molde, Andreassen, Torsheim, & Pallesen, 2014).

These trends have been accompanied by observations about the changing nature of drug consumption across societies. In particular, concerns have been raised about the normalisation of drug consumption, especially among supplements, illicit and performance enhancing drugs. Supplementation plays a significant role in normalising expectations of the need for drugs in response to everyday activity, whether minimising the potential length of unpredictable minor illnesses (e.g. Vitamin C and colds), overcoming performance decrements (e.g. responding to fatigue with ginkgo biloba) or performance enhancement (e.g. fish oil to enhance cognitive function). The normalising effect of illicit drugs is seen in the belief that such drugs are an unremarkable part of society (Aldridge, Measham, & Williams, 2011) and can be seen as an integral part of socialising (e.g. Duff, 2005). Illicit drugs are then being integrated into everyday activities (e.g. 'controlled' use of cocaine; Zuffa, Meringolo, & Petrini, 2014). This integration of drugs into normalised activities is also occurring in other specific parts of society, with academics and university students integrating the use of prescription stimulants to enhance academic performance (e.g. Maher, 2008; Schelle *et al.*, 2015). Almost 40 per cent of Australian university students reported that the use of drugs to enhance academic performance (or self-medicate fatigue) was a normal part of their education (Mazanov, Dunn, Connor, & Fielding, 2013).

The normalisation of drugs to enhance performance among otherwise healthy people has been described as 'medically enhanced normality' (Møldrup & Hansen, 2006; Møldrup, Traulsen, & Almarsdóttir, 2003). The evolution of medical drug use saw the transition from curative (e.g. to treat illness) to preventative (e.g. immunisation) treatment. The transition to preventative therapy introduced the idea of medicating the healthy. The next step was the use of drugs to medicate quality of life, such as birth control, sexual function and cosmetic enhancement (e.g. Botox injections). The increasing acceptance of medically enhanced normality can be seen with 'rejuvenation therapy', where drugs like human growth hormone and testosterone are used to medicate physical decline as a result of the ageing process.

Evidence suggests that, unsurprisingly, the control of drugs in sport has little bearing on the way amateur athletes use drugs (Lentillon-Kaestner & Ohl, 2011). For example, when non-elite athletes use drugs, that use is unlikely to be based in an intention to derive an advantage in sport. It would be more common for non-elite athletes to use drugs in an attempt to preserve access to sport. For example, Masters level athletes may use drugs to maintain their ability to participate in sport as they age rather than enhance performance (Henning & Dimeo, 2015). Where drug abuse does occur, it seems to be in ways that represent the problems of misuse and abuse of drugs that potentially threaten the integrity of a society (see Chapters 2 and 3), rather than a direct threat to the integrity of sport (Lentillon-Kaestner & Ohl, 2011).

Non-elite sport and the Code

The anti-doping movement has attempted to leverage the relationship between drugs in sport and drugs in society by introducing a public health discourse. That is, the anti-doping movement has claimed that evidence doping is becoming widespread among non-elite athletes redefines the issue as a looming public health crisis (O'Connor, 2012; Reedie, 2015).

The World Health Organisation defines public health as organised measures to prevent disease, promote health and prolong life at the community or societal level. Drug misuse and abuse lead to physical and psychological dependence that have profound health implications. However, the evidence that doping misuse and abuse is of an order that distinguishes it from other forms of drug misuse or abuse seems a rather extraordinary claim to make given the absence of a reliable epidemiology for doping in elite sport (de Hon, Kuipers, & van Bottenburg, 2015; Petróczi, Mazanov, Nepusz, Backhouse, & Naughton, 2008) let alone the vacuum that is the epidemiology of doping in non-elite sport. Given that most drugs associated with doping have legitimate therapeutic use within the context of sport, and are used to prevent or treat illness and injury, the argument that doping diminishes health can be difficult to sustain. Finally, it is unclear whether doping systematically diminishes life expectancy. While there are well-publicised exceptions (e.g. deaths as a result of misuse of erythropoietin; Parisotto, 2006), it is unclear whether doping can be systematically linked to reduced life expectancy or quality of life across communities in the same way as alcohol, tobacco or heroin. As a result, the claim that doping represents a potential public health crisis appears difficult to sustain in the absence of reliable evidence.

As argued in Chapter 6, critics of anti-doping observe that reconstructing doping as a public health crisis is politically motivated as an attempt to inflate the influence of drug control for sport well beyond the regulatory boundaries of sport (e.g. Waddington, Christiansen, Gleaves, Hoberman, & Møller, 2013). This strategy risks diminishing the role drug control for sport can take in debate around the public health implications of human enhancement technologies more broadly (e.g. mood enhancement and cybernetic prosthetics) on the health of individuals and societies (see Savulescu, ter Meulen, & Kahane, 2011).

Setting aside the conceptual issues, the Code is designed to penetrate all levels of sport, from elite male sport through to membership-based recreational sport. This raises the question whether the Code can be scaled from the controlled context of elite sport to being a genuine societal public health intervention addressing the diverse and unpredictable world of mass participation sport.

Direct translation of the Code from elite sport to non-elite sport would be highly resource intensive. The foundation of the Code is detection-based deterrence (Mazanov & McDermott, 2009), which relies upon investigation and prosecution of ADRV. Hermann and Henneberg (2014) estimate the cost of effective drug testing in elite sport at US$28,600 per athlete. Maennig (2014) estimates drug test-led sanctions cost approximately US$34,650 and that when investigation-led sanctions are taken into account the cost is about US$69,300. These suggest that the costs of detection-based deterrence have been pegged to the capacity for elite male sport to pay. The Texas high school football drug testing programme was expected to cost US$120 per test (US$3 million annual budget testing up to 25,000 athletes per year) (Woolf & Swain, 2014). By its second year (US$6 million allocated) there were 19 drug positives and 137 protocol violations, meaning each sanction cost approximately US$38,400, the majority of which were inconclusive in terms of whether drugs were used. It is unclear whether the programme reduced doping in Texan high school football. Maennig (2014) notes that such estimates miss the indirect costs needed for the administrative architecture that supports drug control in elite sport, such as investment in drug test development, Code updates, awareness activities for the Prohibited List or delivering education programmes. As a result, the actual costs are likely to be more than the estimates.

An obvious answer for non-elite sport is to transfer the costs to participants (e.g. through registration fees) or sponsors, although this would make non-elite sport unaffordable. The attempt to minimise costs and make anti-doping more affordable for non-elite sport has led to innovative approaches being suggested. For example, Henning and Dimeo (2014) suggest 'grass roots' anti-doping through a network of volunteer anti-doping arbitration panels. This creates an extra administrative burden for anti-doping organisations to ensure that volunteers are appropriately qualified to assess and respond to cases, but should enable greater access to the Code at the non-elite level. However, this approach potentially violates the principle of policy harmonisation, as athletes would be exposed to a 'cut down' version of anti-doping which may lead to inequitable outcomes. For example, a non-elite cyclist taking a supplement contaminated with testosterone may be allowed to compete at a Masters event as a result of an inexperienced panel while an elite cyclist taking the same supplement at an Olympic event would be sanctioned. Henning and Dimeo (2014) argue that, rather than applying the same rules to elite and non-elite sport, a drug control germane to non-elite sport is needed.

It is also unclear whether applying the Code to non-elite sport more rigorously would do anything to arrest a doping-led public health crisis. If a doping-led public health crisis emerged, it may be better to respond to it with tools demonstrated to have an impact on health behaviour. For example, the sustained effort to reduce combustible cigarette consumption in the First World using a combination of policy tools (e.g. taxation, education and treatment) has achieved significant successes. With this in mind, the strategy of reconstructing doping as a public health issue may lead to sport ceding control to governments looking to minimise health care costs among its citizens, especially if the use of certain drugs in sport can be demonstrated to reduce health risks (e.g. reduce the risk of sports injury) or improve health outcomes (e.g. increase physical activity rates) (see Chapter 1).

Controlling drugs in non-elite sport

As observed with the arguments presented for women's and children's sport, the challenges facing drug control for non-elite sport are different to those facing elite male sport. Non-elite sport has to manage drugs in a much broader social context, including norms around drugs that may be different to other forms of sport. For example, for non-elite athletes, drugs may have very little to do with the integrity of sport and more to do with a range of other social factors, such as the normalisation of drug use in other aspects of their lives. It is clear that a direct application of the Code to non-elite sport is unlikely to be affordable, suggesting that a different approach to drug control for non-elite sport might be necessary. Pursuing anti-doping at the non-elite level may violate policy harmonisation. Alternatively, drug control in non-elite sport could be addressed as an issue of public health rather than an issue left to the private interests of sport.

Drug control for all sport

It appears that drug control-led integrity management for sport has been predicated on the integrity of elite male sport. As a result, the interests and implications for other versions of sport have been omitted. If drug control is meant to improve the integrity of sport and meet the principles of CSR, sport needs to actively address how drugs affect the integrity of women's, children's and non-elite sport. In terms of drugs generally, sport needs to recognise that its relationship with alcohol is likely to be the greatest threat to its integrity. In terms of anti-doping based drug control, it is clear that the pursuit of equal treatment through policy harmonisation has created significant inequities in the experience of drug control. To some degree, this makes sport seem naive about drug control; that drug use in sport is heterogeneous across demographic categories is a truism in drug control. This raises the question about whether sport should be allowed to learn the lessons of drug control with all the harms to individuals and societies that implies, or whether the harms should be avoided by handing drug control for sport over to public health organisations. It may well be that the integrity of sport would be best served by relinquishing drug control to public health.

References

Aldridge, J., Measham, F., & Williams, L. (2011). *Illegal Leisure Revisited*. East Sussex: Routledge.

Amos, A., & Fridman, S. (2009). Drugs in sport: The legal issues. *Sport in Society*, *12*(3), 356–374.

Aubel, O., & Ohl, F. (2014). An alternative approach to the prevention of doping in cycling. *International Journal of Drug Policy*, *25*(6), 1094–1102.

Backhouse, S. H., Whitaker, L., & Petróczi, A. (2013). Gateway to doping? Supplement use in the context of preferred competitive situations, doping attitude, beliefs, and norms. *Scandinavian Journal of Medicine and Science in Sports*, *23*(2), 244–252.

Baker, J., Koz, D., Kungl, A. M., Fraser-Thomas, J., & Schorer, J. (2013). Staying at the top: Playing position and performance affect career length in professional sport. *High Ability Studies*, *24*(1), 63–76.

BBC (2011). Dutch football club VVV 'signs up' hat-trick toddler. Available at www.bbc.co.uk/news/world-europe-13224130 (accessed 1 March 2016).

Bloodworth, A., & McNamee, M. (2010). Clean Olympians? Doping and anti-doping: The views of talented young British athletes. *International Journal of Drug Policy*, *21*(4), 276–282.

Boyd, A., Van de Velde, S., Pivette, M., Ten Have, M., Florescu, S., O'Neill, S., *et al.* (2015). Gender differences in psychotropic use across Europe: Results from a large cross-sectional, population-based study. *European Psychiatry*, *30*(6), 778–788.

Canadian Centre for Ethics in Sport (2012). Quebec trainer receives five-year ban for trafficking and administration. Available at http://cces.ca/news/quebec-trainer-receives-five-year-ban-trafficking-and-administration (accessed 29 February 2016).

Cooky, C., Dycus, R., & Dworkin, S. L. (2013). 'What makes a woman a woman?' versus 'Our lady of sport': A comparative analysis of the United States and the South African media coverage of Caster Semenya. *Journal of Sport and Social Issues*, *37*(1), 31–56.

Court of Arbitration for Sport (2006). *Sesil Karatancheva v International Tennis Federation (Award)* (Court of Arbitration for Sport, CAS 2006/A/1032, 3 July 2006). Available at: www.doping.nl/media/kb/529/CAS%202006_A_1032%20Sesil%20Karatantcheva%20vs%20ITF%20(OS).pdf (accessed 31 May 2016).

Dawson, D. A., Goldstein, R. B., Saha, T. D., & Grant, B. F. (2015). Changes in alcohol consumption: United States, 2001–2002 to 2012–2013. *Drug and Alcohol Dependence*, *148*(March 2015), 56–61.

de Hon, O., Kuipers, H., & van Bottenburg, M. (2015). Prevalence of doping use in elite sports: A review of numbers and methods. *Sports Medicine*, *45*(1), 57–69.

Duff, C. (2005). Party drugs and party people: Examining the 'normalization' of recreational drug use in Melbourne, Australia. *International Journal of Drug Policy*, *16*(3), 161–170.

Dunn, M., Thomas, J. O., Swift, W., & Burns, L. (2011). Recreational substance use among elite Australian athletes. *Drug and Alcohol Review*, *30*(1), 63–68.

Efverström, A., Ahmadi, N., Bavkström, Å., & Hoff, D. (2014). Anti-doping and legitimacy: An international survey of elite athletes' perceptions. *Performance Enhancement and Health*, *3*(2), 115.

Elbe, A. M., & Overbye, M. (2015). Providing support for athletes with negative experiences during urine doping controls. *Journal of Sport Psychology in Action*, *6*(3), 188–198.

Elbe, A-M., Schlegel, M. M., & Brand, R. (2012). Psychogenic urine retention during doping controls: Consequences for elite athletes. *Performance Enhancement and Health*, *1*(2), 66–74.

Elbe, A. M., Jensen, S. N., Elsborg, P., Wetzke, M., Woldemariam, G. A., Huppertz, B., *et al.* (2016). The urine marker test: An alternative approach to supervised urine collection for doping control. *Sports Medicine*, *46*(1), 15–22.

Flake, C. R., Dufur, M. J., & Moore, E .L. (2013). Advantage men: The sex pay gap in professional tennis. *International Review for the Sociology of Sport*, *48*(3), 366–376.

Frick, B., Humphreys, B. R., & Scheel, F. (2015). Career duration in capital-intensive individualistic sports: Evidence from ski jumping, golf and auto racing. In Rodriguez, P., Kesenne, S., & Koning, R. (Eds.), *The Economics of Competitive Sports* (pp. 152–164). Cheltenham, UK: Edward Elgar.

Fulgoni, V. L., Keast, D. R., & Lieberman, H. R. (2015). Trends in intake and sources of caffeine in the diets of US adults: 2001–2010. *The American Journal of Clinical Nutrition*, *101*(5), 1081–1087.

Fürhapter, C., Blank, C., Leichtfried, V., Mair-Raggautz, M., Müller, D., & Schobersberger, W. (2013). Evaluation of West-Austrian junior athletes' knowledge regarding doping in sports. *Wiener klinische Wochenschrift*, *125*(1–2), 41–49.

Green, K., Nelson, T. F., & Hartmann, D. (2014). Binge drinking and sports participation in college: Patterns among athletes and former athletes. *International Review for the Sociology of Sport*, *49*(3–4), 417–434.

Heggie, V. (2010). Testing sex and gender in sports: Reinventing, reimagining and reconstructing histories. *Endeavour*, *34*(4), 157–163.

Henne, K. E. (2015). *Testing for Athlete Citizenship: Regulating Doping and Sex in Sport*. New Brunswick, NJ: Rutgers University Press.

Henning, A. D., & Dimeo, P. (2014). The complexities of anti-doping violations: A case study of sanctioned cases in all performance levels of USA cycling. *Performance Enhancement and Health*, *3*(3), 159–166.

Henning, A. D., & Dimeo, P. (2015). Questions of fairness and anti-doping in US cycling: The contrasting experiences of professionals and amateurs. *Drugs: Education, Prevention and Policy*, *22*(5), 400–409.

Hermann A., & Henneberg, M. (2014). Anti-doping systems in sports are doomed to fail: A probability and cost analysis. *Journal of Sports Medicine and Doping Studies*, *4*(5).

Hildebrandt, T., Harty, S., & Langenbucher, J. W. (2012). Fitness supplements as a gateway substance for anabolic-androgenic steroid use. *Psychology of Addictive Behaviors*, 26(4), 955–962.

Hoberman, J. (2005). *Testosterone Dreams: Rejuvenation, Aphrodisia, Doping.* Berkeley, CA: University of California Press.

Hubbard, A. (2015). Is rugby the new athletics for doping offenders? Available at: www.insidethegames.biz/articles/1027543/alan-hubbard-is-rugby-the-new-athletics-for-doping-offenders. First published 26 May. (accessed 21 Aug 2015).

IOC (2010). Two Youth Olympic Games athletes disqualified for breaking anti-doping rules in Singapore. Available at: www.olympic.org/content/press-release/press-release-pr65-2010 (accessed 29 August 2015).

IOC (2012). Fact sheet: Youth Olympic Games. Available at: www.olympic. org/documents/Reference_documents_Factsheets/The_Youth_Olympic_Games.pdf (accessed 28 August 2015).

IOC (2014). IOC disqualifies athlete for violating anti-doping rules at the Summer Youth Olympic Games. Available at: www.olympic.org/news/ioc-disqualifies-athlete-for-violating-anti-doping-rules-at-the-summer-youth-olympic-games/240150 (accessed 28 August 2015).

Jordan, S. L., & Naclerio, F. (2014). Ergogenic aids and the female athlete. In Robert-McComb, J., Norman, R., & Zumwalt, M. (Eds.), *The Active Female* (pp. 491–515). New York: Springer.

Karkazis, K., Jordan-Young, R., Davis, G., & Camporesi, S. (2012). Out of bounds? A critique of the new policies on hyperandrogenism in elite female sports. *American Journal of Bioethics*, 12(7), 3–16.

Kelly, B. C., Wells, B. E., Pawson, M., LeClair, A., & Parsons, J. T. (2014). Combinations of prescription drug misuse and illicit drugs among young adults. *Addictive Behaviors*, 39(5), 941–944.

Kenny, K., & Bell, E. (2011). Representing the successful managerial body. In E. L. Jaenes, D. Knights, & P. Yancey Martin (Eds.), *Handbook of Gender, Work and Organization*. Chichester, UK: Wiley.

Keyes, K. M., Li, G., & Hasin, D. S. (2011). Birth cohort effects and gender differences in alcohol epidemiology: A review and synthesis. *Alcoholism: Clinical and Experimental Research*, 35(12), 2101–2112.

Korvajarvi, P. (2011). Practicing gender neutrality in organisations. In E. L. Jeanes, D. Knights, & P. Yancey Martin (Eds.), *Handbook of Gender, Work and Organizations* (pp. 231–244). Chichester, UK: Wiley.

Kwan, M., Bobko, S., Faulkner, G., Donnelly, P., & Cairney, J. (2014). Sport participation and alcohol and illicit drug use in adolescents and young adults: A systematic review of longitudinal studies. *Addictive Behaviors*, 39(3), 497–506.

Lenskyj, H. J. (2003). *Out on the Field: Gender, Sport and Sexuality.* Toronto: Women's Press.

Lentillon-Kaestner, V., & Carstairs, C. (2010). Doping use among young elite cyclists: A qualitative psychosociological approach. *Scandinavian Journal of Medicine and Science in Sports*, 20(2), 336–345.

Lentillon-Kaestner, V., & Ohl, F. (2011). Can we measure accurately the prevalence of doping? *Scandinavian Journal of Medicine and Science in Sports*, 21(6), e132-e142.

Lentillon-Kaestner, V., Hagger, M. S., & Hardcastle, S. (2012). Health and doping in elite-level cycling. *Scandinavian Journal of Medicine and Science in Sports*, 22(5), 596–606.

Lisha, N. E., & Sussman, S. (2010). Relationship of high school and college sports participation with alcohol, tobacco, and illicit drug use: A review. *Addictive Behaviors*, 35(5), 399–407.

Maennig, W. (2014). Inefficiency of the anti-doping system: Cost reduction proposals. *Substance Use and Misuse*, 49(9), 1201–1205.

Magdalinksi, T. (2009). *Sport, Technology and the Body*. Abingdon: Routledge.

Maher, B. (2008). Poll results: look who's doping. *Nature*, 452(7188), 674–675.

Mazanov, J., & McDermott, V. (2009). The case for a social science of drugs in sport. *Sport in Society*, 12(3), 276–295.

Mazanov, J., Petróczi, A., Bingham, J., & Holloway, A. (2008). Towards an empirical model of performance enhancing supplement use: A pilot study among high performance UK athletes. *Journal of Science and Medicine in Sport*, 11(2), 185–190.

Mazanov, J., Dunn, M., Connor, J., & Fielding, M. L. (2013). Substance use to enhance academic performance among Australian university students. *Performance Enhancement and Health*, 2(3), 110–118.

Mazanov, J., Backhouse, S., Connor, J., Hemphill, D., & Quirk, F. (2014). Athlete support personnel and anti-doping: Knowledge, attitudes, and ethical stance. *Scandinavian Journal of Medicine and Science in Sports*, 24(5), 846–856.

Mazanov, J., Hemphill, D., Connor, J., Quirk, F., & Backhouse, S. H. (2015). Australian athlete support personnel lived experience of anti-doping. *Sport Management Review*, 18(2), 218–230.

McGannon, K. R., Gonsalves, C. A., Schinke, R. J., & Busanich, R. (2015). Negotiating motherhood and athletic identity: A qualitative analysis of Olympic athlete mother representations in media narratives. *Psychology of Sport and Exercise*, 20(2015), 51–59.

Møldrup, C., & Hansen, R. (2006). Public acceptance of drug use for non-disease conditions. *Current Medical Research and Opinion*, 22(4), 775–780.

Møldrup, C., Traulsen, J. M., & Almarsdóttir, A. B. (2003). Medically-enhanced normality: An alternative perspective on the use of medicines for non-medical purposes. *International Journal of Pharmacy Practice*, 11(4), 243–249.

Ng, M., Freeman, M. K., Fleming, T. D., Robinson, M., Dwyer-Lindgren, L., Thomson, B., *et al.* (2014). Smoking prevalence and cigarette consumption in 187 countries, 1980–2012. *JAMA*, 311(2), 183–192.

O'Connor, P. (2012). Doping is now a public health issue, conference told. Available at: http://uk.reuters.com/article/us-doping-health-idUSBRE88L06E20120922 (accessed 29 February 2016).

Ohl, F., Finocouer, B., Lentillon-Kaestnar, V., Defrance, J., & Brissonneau, C. (2015). The socialization of young cyclists and the culture of doping. *International Review for the Sociology of Sport*, 50(7), 865–882.

Palmer, F. R., & Leberman, S. I. (2009). Elite athletes as mothers: Managing multiple sport identities. *Sport Management Review*, 12(4), 241–254.

Papadopoulos, F. C., Skalkidis, I., Parkkari, J., & Petridou, E. (2006). Doping use among tertiary education students in six developed countries. *European Journal of Epidemiology*, 21(4), 307–313.

Parisotto, R. (2006). *Bloodsports. The Inside Dope on Drugs in Sport*. Prahran, Australia: Hardie Grant.

Paulozzi, L. J., Jones, C., Mack, K., & Rudd, R. (2011). Vital signs: overdoses of prescription opioid pain relievers – United States, 1999–2008. *Morbidity and Mortality Weekly Report, 60*(43), 1487–1492.

Penolazzi, B., Natale, V., Leone, L., & Russo, P. M. (2012). Individual differences affecting caffeine intake. Analysis of consumption behaviours for different times of day and caffeine sources. *Appetite, 58*(3), 971–977.

Petróczi, A., Mazanov, J., & Naughton, D. P. (2011). Inside athletes' minds: Preliminary results from a pilot study on mental representation of doping and potential implications for anti-doping. *Substance Abuse Treatment, Prevention and Policy, 6*(10).

Petróczi, A., Mazanov, J., Nepusz, T., Backhouse, S. H., & Naughton, D. P. (2008). Comfort in big numbers: Does over-estimation of doping prevalence in others indicate self-involvement? *Journal of Occupational Medicine and Toxicology, 3*(19).

Pfister, G. (2010). Women in sport-gender relations and future perspectives. *Sport in Society, 13*(2), 234–248.

Piñeiro, B., Correa, J. B., Simmons, V. N., Harrell, P. T., Menzie, N. S., Unrod, M., et al. (2016). Gender differences in use and expectancies of e-cigarettes: Online survey results. *Addictive Behaviors, 52*(1), 91–97.

Pitsch, W., & Emrich, E. (2012). The frequency of doping in elite sport: Results of a replication study. *International Review for the Sociology of Sport, 47*(5), 559–580.

Reedie, C. (2015). WADA President: 'Combatting doping now as important to society as it is to sport'. Available at: www.wada-ama.org/en/media/news/2015-02/wada-president-combatting-doping-now-as-important-to-society-as-it-is-to-sport (accessed 29 February 2016).

Sagoe, D., Molde, H., Andreassen, C. S., Torsheim, T., & Pallesen, S. (2014). The global epidemiology of anabolic-androgenic steroid use: A meta-analysis and meta-regression analysis. *Annals of Epidemiology, 24*(5), 383–398.

Savulescu, J., ter Meulen, R., & Kahane, G. (Eds.). (2011). *Enhancing Human Capacities*. Chichester, UK: Wiley.

Schaal, K., Tafflet, M., Nassif, H., Thibault, V., Pichard, C., Alcotte, M., et al. (2011). Psychological balance in high level athletes: Gender-based differences and sport-specific patterns. *PloS ONE, 6*(5), e19007.

Schelle, K. J., Olthof, B. M., Reintjes, W., Bundt, C., Gusman-Vermeer, J., & van Mil, A. C. (2015). A survey of substance use for cognitive enhancement by university students in the Netherlands. *Frontiers in Systems Neuroscience, 9*(10).

Schneider, A. (2010). On the definition of 'women' in the sport context. In P. Davis and C. Weaving (Eds.), *Handbook of Gender, Work and Organization*. Chichester, UK: Wiley.

Simoni-Wastila, L. (2000). The use of abusable prescription drugs: The role of gender. *Journal of Women's Health and Gender-Based Medicine, 9*(3), 289–297.

Stambulova, N., Stephan, Y., & Jäphag, U. (2007). Athletic retirement: A cross-national comparison of elite French and Swedish athletes. *Psychology of Sport and Exercise, 8*(1), 101–118.

Stewart, B., & Smith, A. C. (2008). Drug use in sport implications for public policy. *Journal of Sport and Social Issues, 32*(3), 278–298.

Suzic Lazic, J., Dikic, N., Radivojevic, N., Mazic, S., Radovanovic, D., Mitrovic, N., *et al.* (2011). Dietary supplements and medications in elite sport – polypharmacy or real need? *Scandinavian Journal of Medicine and Science in Sports*, 21(2), 260–267.

Teetzel, S., & Mazzucco, M. (2014). Minor problems: The recognition of young athletes in the development of international anti-doping policies. *International Journal of the History of Sport*, 31(8), 914–933.

United Nations Office on Drugs and Crime (2015). *World Drug Report 2015*. New York: United Nations.

Waddington, I., Christiansen, A. V., Gleaves, J., Hoberman, J., & Møller, V. (2013). Recreational drug use and sport: Time for a WADA rethink? *Performance Enhancement and Health*, 2(2), 41–47.

Weaving, C., & Teetzel, S. (2014). Getting jacked and burning fat: Examining doping and gender stereotypes in Canadian university sport. *Journal of Intercollegiate Sport*, 7(2), 198–217.

Whitehead, A. (2005). A man to violence: How masculinity may work as a dynamic risk factor. *The Howard Journal*, 44(4), 411–422.

Woolf, J., & Swain, P. (2014). Androgenic anabolic steroid policy and high school sports: Results from a policy Delphi study. *International Journal of Sport Policy and Politics*, 6(1), 89–106.

World Health Organisation (2014). *Global Status Report on Alcohol and Health 2014*. Geneva: World Health Organisation.

Yusko, D. A., Buckman, J. F., White, H. R., & Pandina, R. J. (2008). Alcohol, tobacco, illicit drugs, and performance enhancers: A comparison of use by college student athletes and non-athletes. *Journal of American College Health*, 57(3), 281–290.

Zuffa, G., Meringolo, P., & Petrini, F. (2014). Cocaine users and self-regulation mechanisms. *Drugs and Alcohol Today*, 14(4), 194–206.

Chapter 12

Second generation drug control for sport

Drug control-led integrity management for sport has proven to be a difficult undertaking. Part of the difficulty lies in the privileged structural anti-doping hegemony (see Chapter 3 and 4), which inhibits the capacity for top-down (e.g. alternative paradigms) or bottom-up (e.g. market led responses) innovation in the management of drugs in sport (Mazanov, 2014). Innovation in sports drug control has so far come as conceptual policy discussion such as Stewart and Smith's (2014) manifesto. These discussions tend to omit detail of what the management of drugs in sport might look like under policy alternatives, failing to deliver an administrative framework for 'second generation drug control' (Mazanov & Connor, 2010).

An attempt is made to begin operationalising harm-minimisation as the most mature of the alternative policy approaches emerging from the drugs in sport debate (see Chapter 4). A set of assumptions that guide the alternative are established, followed by how those assumptions might be put into practice exploiting existing systemic governance mechanisms introduced to give effect to anti-doping (see Chapter 7). The implications of this approach are then discussed. Recognising that drug control is always a matter of trading harms (Weatherburn, 2008), the potentially negative outcomes arising from the implementation of harm-minimisation are considered. This consideration points out that, like anti-doping, a harm-minimisation approach to managing drugs in sport leads to a set of wicked problems. In doing so, it raises an important question about which of the two approaches is more likely to better manage integrity for sport.

Harm-minimisation

The discussion of harm-minimisation offered in Chapter 4 is expanded slightly to facilitate the discussion. Harm-minimisation recognises that no approach to drug control is going to eliminate drug misuse or abuse, or the harms that come with drug misuse or abuse (see Chapter 2). As such, it never seeks to 'win the war on drugs' (see Chapter 3). Instead harm-minimisation looks to determine which harms have the greatest impact and then strategise how to minimise those harms. Harm-minimisation arguments posit that supply and demand approaches to drug control (e.g. interdiction and criminal sanction) create more harms in responding to drugs than other approaches might (e.g. blood-borne viruses caused by sharing 'dirty' needles, sending drug addicts to prison, and poverty). Prioritising harm reduction requires a different approach, usually based on treating drug misuse or abuse.

The definition of health and the harms that are minimised are central to the discussion. Mazanov (2016) argues that narrow Western medicalised views of health in the context of sports drug control fail to capture the multitude of ways health is understood across social contexts. A pluralistic approach to health and well-being is therefore taken, such that a harm-minimisation approach to drug control for sport needs to respond to drug consumption that harms physical, psychological, social or spiritual health and well-being.

A harm reduction focused drug control programme for sport, drawn from the manifesto offered by Stewart and Smith (2014), may have as its overarching aim: 'Protecting the health and well-being of participants during and after their sporting careers through the use of drugs for prevention of illness or injury, and treatment in cases of drug misuse or abuse.' From this point of view, participants should be able to use drugs that protect their long-term health and well-being from sport. For example, if the use of erythropoietin can be demonstrated to protect the long-term health of professional road cyclists they would be able to use that drug. The threshold test that triggers a response is when a drug has been deemed to have been misused or abused such that it threatens the health or well-being of an athlete.

Implementation of harm-minimisation

Implementing harm-minimisation uses the overarching aim to establish a framework for classifying drug use, misuse and abuse as the basis for drug control, whether the sports drug matrix (see Chapter 2) or some other approach. This is then supported by drug testing to establish whether athletes meet the health and well-being threshold for fitness to compete (Dunn, 2013; Lippi, Franchini, & Guidi, 2008; Mazanov, 2016). Where athletes are deemed unfit to compete they are denied access to events until they can demonstrate they are fit to compete. Thus, like the World Anti-Doping Code (the Code), the harm-minimisation approach argued here has drug testing as its central mechanism.

Drug control

The fulcrum for drug control is detecting differences between drug use, misuse and abuse. The basis for what is considered safe or unsafe can use Phase I–IV clinical trials to develop reference criteria for distinguishing use from misuse or abuse. This could include safety trials within specific sporting contexts (e.g. contact sports), consistent with trials looking to establish 'off-label' use of drugs with different health conditions (e.g. aspirin for heart conditions) or populations (e.g. children).

Drug control could also look to the effects of drugs rather than inferring their presence or absence. For example, rather than attempting to detect whether erythropoietin has been used to stimulate red blood cell production, Savulescu, Foddy, and Clayton (2004) propose the primary concern should be whether an athlete crosses a threshold haematocrit (a measure of red blood cell concentration) that increases their relative risk of morbidity or mortality. When assessing the ethical harms of anti-doping against harm-minimisation, Savulescu *et al.* argue that testing the health implications of a drug's effects is an ethically defensible means of drug control.

Misuse or abuse can then be defined as exceeding evidence-based safety limits. Where an athlete crosses the threshold they are deemed to be unfit to compete. These limits can be liberal or conservative. A liberal limit might be set where only large doses lead to negative health consequences (e.g. caffeine), and a conservative limit where little is known about how a drug works in the sporting context. A drug can be banned by declaring its presence compromises the health and well-being of an athlete, rendering them unfit to compete until it is completely eliminated from their system. For example, heroin may be banned given the significant health and well-being implications that the drug has.

Drug testing

The drug testing approach exploits a combination of Bird and Wagner's (1997) diary approach and the biological passport (Saugy, Lundby, & Robinson, 2014; Sottas, Robinson, Rabin, & Saugy, 2011). Accepting Bird and Wagner's argument in support of a diary, elite athletes aged 15 years and over (the age at which sport deems athletes are able to consent to anti-doping; see Chapter 11) are required to maintain a public diary of all drugs they have used under the supervision (e.g. countersignature) of appropriately qualified personnel (e.g. sports physicians). This diary is supported by independent accredited laboratories conducting sample collection and analysis. The drug testing procedure could exploit advances in urinary dye markers (see Chapter 11) or through encouraging pharmaceutical companies to include markers that make the detection of drugs less resource intensive (see Chapters 7 and 8). Athletes may elect to be tested more frequently (e.g. monthly). The diary and independent testing enable a version of out-of-competition testing through ongoing audit by a central body (see below).

Entry to elite events is contingent upon athletes submitting to a drug test whose results are compared against their diary and independent testing. Where the drug test results are consistent with what has been recorded in the diary (e.g. acknowledging measurement error), athletes are permitted to compete at the event. In effect, the drug test is an assurance the athlete is fit to compete, at least in terms of drug use.

Non-elite athletes and athletes under 15 years maintain a private diary supervised by a general medicine practitioner (e.g. family general practitioner) and local pathology laboratories for events that require the diary and test for entry. For example, a local fun run may choose to avoid testing whereas a Masters tournament may wish to control entry based on testing.

Athletes fail the drug test in one of three ways. The first is when the pattern of results from the drug diary suggests drug misuse or abuse, along the same lines as the biological passport (Saugy et al., 2014). The second is that the results exceed a predetermined limit aimed at protecting athlete health and well-being. The third is the detection of something that is absent from their diary, which is primarily intended as a conservative response to novel drugs with unknown health and well-being implications, but also creates a structural incentive to disclose which drugs an athlete has used. A test failure triggers an evaluation by a panel of professionals qualified to assess the test results in terms of whether the failure constitutes a health risk. The test failure is then supported by a report outlining the opinion of the panel. This opinion can be appealed to central sports drug control organisations (see below).

Disqualification and treatment

Where an athlete fails a drug test for a reason deemed to constitute a health and/or well-being risk, they are disqualified from competing in events as being unfit for competition. Once an athlete has been disqualified from an event, they are unable to return for that event even if subsequent testing shows they have returned to normal. For example, an athlete demonstrating a spike immediately before the Olympics would be denied entry even if their levels subsequently return to normal by the time their event had commenced. This creates an incentive for athletes to ensure their drug use is within prescribed limits.

Athletes are allowed to return to competition once the levels return to the established limits. This approach means that the length of disqualification can be highly variable. It is within the realms of possibility for this system to see an athlete return to competition within days or weeks, or for an athlete to never return if they are unable to use rather than misuse or abuse drugs to support their sporting ambitions. Where drug testing reveals anomalous results that threaten health (e.g. drug abuse), as already happens in men's professional sports in the United States (see Chapter 9), they can be compelled to receive treatment as a condition of returning to competition (cf. D'Angelo & Tamburrini, 2010). For example, an athlete abusing sleeping tablets to cope with competition (Dunn, 2014) may be referred for treatment to help them cope with sport more effectively.

Harm-minimisation administration

The aim of this section is to provide an indication of how the administration might work rather than provide an exhaustive account. Given the length of the Code and the administrative complexities of anti-doping organisations it would be inappropriate to attempt to deal with the breadth of issues in this chapter. That significant administrative implications need to be teased out is acknowledged, and represents another aspect for debate in establishing second generation drug control-led integrity management for sport.

Giving effect to harm-minimisation would require tailoring of the existing anti-doping architecture rather than replacement. Conventions and organisations refocus to become sports drug organisations to achieve the overarching aim of protecting athlete health and welfare, notionally titled the World Sports Drug Code (WSDC). In the first instance, WADA can become the World Sports Drug Agency (WSDA) to establish and administer the WSDC (Mazanov, 2013). Following the criticisms of democratisation in sport (see Chapter 7), the board structure needs to include stakeholders across the breadth of sport, including athletes, pharmaceutical companies, the media, volunteers and fans. Boards must also be structured to ensure that the interests of non-Olympic, women's, children's and non-elite sport are represented (see Chapter 11). Funding can be drawn from a system of contributions driven by international conventions, by developing a fee structure for membership and/or accreditation, or marketising membership (see Chapter 5).

Like WADA, the WSDA leadership role is defined as a lead policy agency that works towards:

- establishing, updating and disseminating the criteria for safe drug use in sport,
- developing model policy and WSDC interactions with other legal frameworks (e.g. human rights),
- working to achieve policy harmonisation across sports and jurisdictions,
- accreditation of sports drug control laboratories,
- co-ordinating education about use, misuse and abuse of drugs in sport (e.g. athletes, support personnel and review panels), and
- being the final appeal in response to disqualification decisions.

Following the anti-doping architecture, domestic drug control for sport would be handled by National or Regional Sports Drug Agencies (NSDA and RSDA, respectively). These organisations would focus on implementation, including:

- quality control of events claiming WSDC compliance,
- co-ordinating accredited testing,
- ensuring review panels are appropriately qualified,
- education about use, misuse and abuse of drugs in sport, and
- hearing disqualification appeals.

Individual events would be responsible for establishing whether they are sports drug control compliant. Events may choose to be sports drug control compliant on the basis of level of sport (e.g. control would negatively impact participation), marketing (e.g. as part of a broader marketing strategy) (see Chapter 10), or a requirement stipulated in broadcast or sponsorship contracts. Events could 'buy in' drug control from their domestic agency, or set up their own drug control system for domestic accreditation.

Transitioning from the Code

Transitioning from the Code to any alternative approach to drug control is going to be a significant undertaking for sports managers and administrators. Retaining the focus on drug testing means that much of the architecture used to administer the Code can be translated to harm-minimisation. The aim here is to identify that transitioning from the Code is feasible, and to highlight some of the core issues that need to be addressed in doing so.

For this discussion it is worth noting that the Code had a long gestation (see Chapter 3). While it may be hoped that a second generation response would be implemented more rapidly than the 70 or so years taken by anti-doping, the change would still take decades rather than years to manifest fully.

Institutional change

Institutional change seeks support from stakeholders assuming leadership roles in drug control for sport (see Chapter 7). The inertia in international treaties and conventions means support at this level is necessary. There may also be political resistance from the United Nations more broadly which traditionally takes a conservative 'war on drugs' approach to drug control (cf. Bewley-Taylor, 2003, 2005). The International Olympic Committee and governments who contribute to WADA would also need to be convinced of the change. This presents a particular problem for governments where harm-minimisation may be inconsistent with domestic 'zero tolerance' drug control policies. Support from sporting federations and governing bodies may be sluggish given the inertia associated with the strength of anti-doping as a marketing device (see Chapter 10).

Influencing such a diverse group of organisations means harm-minimisation needs robust arguments that align with the vested interests of those groups (Mazanov, Huybers, & Connor, 2012). For example, concerns around supervised drug use can be argued in terms of public health (reduced overall drug harms to society and individuals) and evidence-based medicine on treatment based approaches. Concerns around the impact on performance can be argued as a more efficient version of drug control that mitigates drug-based performance inequities consistent with increasing acceptability of drug use to enhance quality of life (see Chapter 11).

Market driven change

Market driven change emerges where individual domestic sports adopt harm-minimisation, which then compels institutions to change. This follows the market-based policy experiment logic argued by Mazanov (2014).

Three critical milestones are needed for market driven change to have an effect. The first is that the initial implementation of harm-minimisation should be in a sport with a non-Code based approach to drug control, such as bodybuilding or entertainment wrestling. The first mover would need enough resource reserves to sustain innovation costs such as developing the administrative architecture and risks to revenue from government funding, sponsors or broadcasters. The market then responds to the alternative drug control in terms of audiences (attendance and broadcast) and sponsors, which would send a clear signal on market drug control preferences for sport. If the signal is positive other sports may adopt the alternative approach, perhaps in less mainstream participation sports such as extreme sports (e.g. mixed martial arts) or chess.

The second milestone is adoption by a mainstream non-Olympic sport, such as American Football, rugby (league or union), cricket or tenpin bowling. A critical mass of mainstream non-Olympic sports then creates market pressure towards the alternative.

The final milestone would be the adoption of harm-minimisation by Olympic sports at the expense of their Olympic status; cycling, football (soccer), ice hockey or tennis are candidates given their revenue base means they are likely to survive independently of a relationship with the Olympic movement. Such a market driven change would force institutional responses to align with practice rather than policy. Failure of, for example, the Olympics to respond to the revealed drug control preferences of the market by abandoning sports which renege on Code compliance would see it cease to be viable as a global sporting mega-event.

Operationalising harm-minimisation

Operationalising harm-minimisation to manage drugs in sport has been presented as an adaptation of the anti-doping policy. This has been done for two reasons. The first is to acknowledge the crucial contribution of anti-doping. Adapting the existing architecture recognises and leverages the important contributions and lessons of anti-doping as first generation drug control for sport (Mazanov & Connor, 2010). To replace anti-doping in its entirety would waste the tremendous amount of human and financial resources invested in establishing drug control for sport. The second is that it makes the process of changing the way drugs are managed in sport less daunting. While used to promote harm-minimisation here, it also creates the possibility of considering how the anti-doping administrative architecture might be adapted to give effect to other alternative approaches to sports drug control (see Chapter 4).

Harm-minimisation and the challenges of anti-doping

Harm-minimisation approaches to drug control for sport have been set up in opposition to or contrast with anti-doping (Mazanov, 2014). This means that sports drug harm-minimisation has been constructed to directly address some of the problems arising from anti-doping while preserving some features. As a result, the harm-minimisation approach offered here continues to protect the ideals of health, fairness and equity in sport set out in the Code, just in a different way. The auditing of athlete health and well-being clearly meets the first criterion. The notion of 'fairness' might actually be improved with increasing interest in sports drug innovation. Elite athletes and sports programmes would have access to each other's drug diaries, while non-elite athletes would be controlled relative to known safety limits. Performance implications may therefore be a function of pharmacogenetic interactions, which could be argued to represent another expression of human interaction with technology (e.g. pole vaults, shark skin swim suits or laser eye surgery). Of course, the 'unlevel playing field' would exist as wealthy countries would have more resources to invest in finding the optimal mix between the genetic potential of athletes and pharmaceutical technologies; drug control will never be able to resolve this issue. While there would still be a significant cost burden associated with testing that may have implications for investment in non-elite sport (Henning & Dimeo, 2014, 2015), the improving knowledge base around safe use of drugs could see non-elite sport become less vulnerable to misuse and abuse.

The harm-minimisation approach offered also addresses a number of inequities arising from anti-doping's focus on non-elite, non-male sport (see Chapter 11). Drug testing fundamentally changes, with athletes able to choose, for the most part, when and where they are tested. The rights of the child are more certain with an established minimum age for consent consistent with the IOC position on when a child is able to understand the implications of drug control, although an empirically determined age of consent would be preferable. The potential distress at refusing a drug test is reduced as a refusal only has implications for a single event rather than a period of exclusion. Removal of sanctions for elite and professional athletes should alleviate conflicts of interest arising from drug control. While the interpretation of the test results may be open to debate, the test results and their measurement error would represent objective facts used both in establishing and appealing a decision. The issue of gender equity in sanctions would become irrelevant.

Unlike anti-doping, the proposed approach explicitly acknowledges that drugs are a fundamental part of sports culture and seeks to work in sympathy with rather than oppose that culture through prohibition. Cultural norms around drug use would be shaped by transparent independently derived and communicated health standards rather than social norms derived through speculation on why a drug has been prohibited (Milot, 2014). Of course, it would be naive to assume that this would yield universal functional drug cultures in sport, as social processes would inevitably lead to resistance (e.g. privileging information from personal networks over official information). However, such resistance would occur irrespective of the underlying drug policy.

Debate would shift from performance to health and well-being implications of a drug. For example, the debate around the paradox where marijuana, as a performance diminishing drug, is prohibited while caffeine, a performance enhancing drug, would simply disappear (see Chapter 4). Debate would continue to be nuanced and polarising under the ongoing renegotiation of what is understood to constitute health and well-being in sport and society. From the harm-minimisation point of view, this is a functional debate as it focuses on minimising drug-based health and well-being harms arising from sport.

Potential wicked problems for harm-minimisation

While harm-minimisation directly addresses some of the problems arising from the Code, the trading of harms means that the attempt to solve one set of problems creates a new set of problems. The discussion draws on Mazanov's (2016) critique of harm-minimisation. Assuming transitioning away from the Code takes decades, some of these issues may well be resolved by the time an attempt to move harm-minimisation from concept to practice emerges.

Risk of abuse

An immediate critique of harm-minimisation is that use increases the risk of misuse or abuse. The provision of information on prescribed safety limits of drugs may be misinterpreted by some as indicating that a drug is 'safe'. For example, naive drug users may fail to grasp the notion of dose-response and fall into misuse with simple heuristics like 'one is good, ten must be better'. This raises a risk of misuse or abuse, although whether this is the same, better or worse than that experienced under the Code remains to be seen.

The risk of misuse, especially at non-elite levels, may increase by taxing the knowledge base of supervising medical practitioners. While it may be reasonable to expect sports physicians (specialist medical practitioners with post-graduate qualifications) to have expert insight into how drugs work in sport, it would add another knowledge burden to general medicine practitioners already required to maintain currency on an enormous range of medical conditions. One answer may be to develop a more stringent accreditation among the cadre of 'sports doctors' (general practice with an interest in sport), which potentially inflates the bureaucracy and a consequent increase in costs.

Ethical resistance

Providing information about how best to use drugs may prove to be ethically challenging for those who believe that such technologies impugn sport as a virtuous activity. This is likely to lead to resistance among those groups, similar to those advocates of harm-minimisation currently engaged in ethical resistance to the Code. While this may create problems in terms of the politics of sport and sports ethics, the inherent value is that ongoing critical reflection caused by resistance ensures drug control for sport continues to evolve beyond both anti-doping and harm-minimisation.

Prioritising secondary prevention

The harm-minimisation approach articulated prioritises secondary prevention, or seeking to minimise potential or actual damage through disqualification and treatment. Arguing harm-minimisation is primary prevention (e.g. preventing harm through educating athletes about safe use) is more difficult to defend given the overarching focus on responding to drug misuse or abuse.

Assuming harm-minimisation prioritises secondary prevention, there are significant risks of unknown long-term health implications arising from the combination of drugs. Medical science goes to some lengths to explore which drugs can be used in combination, and where use of one drug contraindicates use of another. Given the enthusiasm for both breadth of consumption and willingness to consume experimental drugs under the Code (see Chapter 8), it remains to be seen whether the sports pharmacopoeia athletes are willing to consider would expand in harmful ways under harm-minimisation. The potentially infinite combinations of drugs used by athletes could pose a significant threat to health that would tax the boundaries of knowledge for both sports medicine and sports science. This suggests a transfer of costs from the development of drug tests to increasing the costs towards understanding how drugs interact within the human organism. Of course, redirecting medical research funding from developing drug tests to better understanding drug interactions may be considered a better investment. The fact that harm-minimisation introduces such arguments indicates that the prioritisation of secondary prevention may be a wicked problem.

Coercion

A core ethical foundation to the Code is that it seeks to give athletes the choice to remain 'drug free', protecting athletes from coercion to use drugs (Kirkwood, 2009; Miah, 2004; Schneider, 2004). That is, athletes being forced to use drugs to be competitive where they otherwise would have remained abstinent, especially at the elite level. Arguably, despite the Code, athletes are already coerced into using drugs omitted from the Prohibited List. As noted in Chapters 1 and 3, the nature of modern sport suggests athletes no longer have a choice of whether drugs form part of their sporting practice, only a choice of which drugs to use. The wicked problem that emerges for harm-minimisation is whether it increases the risk of coercion. This issue needs to be developed to determine the boundaries of how harm-minimisation drug control works in the sporting context and whether that is a more or less acceptable harm relative to the Code.

Drug diaries and drug testing

A vulnerability of the proposed approach is the integrity of the drug diaries. Bird and Wagner (1997) caveat their advocacy for the diary with those who intentionally seek to undermine its intent (e.g. falsified entries, undetectable drugs or timing the effect of drugs to peak after the entry test). Further, the incentives for suppliers to develop undetectable drugs would remain. This means that the inefficiencies associated with the 'doping arms race' would continue as a feature of any drug control system that relied on drug testing (see Mazanov & McDermott, 2009). It is in this space that organised crime would continue to flourish, although hopefully in a market of significantly lower value. This is effectively the same problem faced by the Code and indeed any drug control that relies on drug testing.

The wickedness of harm-minimisation

The wicked problems of harm-minimisation give a clear indication that no approach to drug control in sport is going to resolve current or future problems. Instead, the potential wicked problems observed for a harm-minimisation approach point to the clear need to manage drugs by experimenting with different policies and systems that can adapt to the evolving role of drugs in sport and society.

Second generation drug control for sport and sports integrity

Harm-minimisation is by no means a drug control-led integrity management panacea for sport. Implementing harm-minimisation would bring with it very difficult challenges for sport, including convincing producers and consumers their rules- and values-based expectations are met under the policy. For example, harm-minimisation asks the broader question about what is meant by integrity in sport by challenging whether the 'fairness' or 'level playing field' constructions of integrity are relevant to the question of drug control. However, sport is willing to do difficult things to win the trust of producers and consumers, demonstrated by the sustained effort that led to the introduction of the anti-doping policy and its supporting administration.

In terms of the implications for the integrity of sport, discussion of harm-minimisation shows that, despite the anti-doping hegemony, policy alternatives do exist and that they can be implemented. The threat to integrity management for sport is perhaps the apparent unwillingness to consider alternative ways to construct integrity for sport, or preventing the evolution of sports integrity management by consolidating behind a single approach. While sport is willing to do difficult things to win the trust of producers and consumers, it has also been reluctant to change once an approach has been taken. As argued in Chapter 10, it will probably take another crisis before sport is willing to evolve its approach to integrity management. As Pound, McLaren, and Younger (2015) assert, it is naive to think that athletics is the only sport having difficulty meeting its obligations under the Code. If true, it is only a matter of time before the concatenation of doping-related scandals mount to create the crisis that provokes drug control-led integrity management for sport to evolve.

The need for adaptability serves as a valuable insight for integrity management more generally. The key here is that, rather than scrap an entire administrative system, the administrative architecture designed to promote one version of integrity can be redeployed should rules- and/or values-based expectations change. While doing so is likely to reveal new concerns, this is the process by which both the understanding and practice of integrity and integrity management evolve.

References

Bewley-Taylor, D. R. (2003). Challenging the UN drug control conventions: Problems and possibilities. *International Journal of Drug Policy, 14*(2), 171–179.

Bewley-Taylor, D. R. (2005). Emerging policy contradictions between the United Nations drug control system and the core values of the United Nations. *International Journal of Drug Policy, 16*(6), 423–431.

Bird, E. J., & Wagner, G. G. (1997). Sport as a common property resource. A solution to the dilemmas of doping. *Journal of Conflict Resolution, 41*(6), 749–766.

D'Angelo, C., & Tamburrini, C. (2010). Addict to win? A different approach to doping. *Journal of Medical Ethics, 36*(11), 700–707.

Dunn, M. (2013). Commentary: Ending the ban on recreational substance use in sport: And then what? *Performance Enhancement and Health, 2*(2), 64–65.

Dunn, M. (2014). The importance of understanding motives for prescription substance use and misuse in sport. *Performance Enhancement & Health, 3*(2), 102–104.

Henning, A. D., & Dimeo, P. (2014). The complexities of anti-doping violations: A case study of sanctioned cases in all performance levels of USA cycling. *Performance Enhancement and Health, 3*(3), 159–166.

Henning, A. D., & Dimeo, P. (2015). Questions of fairness and anti-doping in US cycling: The contrasting experiences of professionals and amateurs. *Drugs: Education, Prevention and Policy, 22*(5), 400–409.

Kirkwood, K. (2009). Considering harm reduction as the future of doping control policy in international sport. *Quest, 61*(2), 180–190.

Lippi, G., Franchini, M., & Guidi, G. C. (2008). Doping in competition or doping in sport? *British Medical Bulletin, 86*(1), 95–107.

Mazanov, J. (2013). *Vale* WADA, *ave* 'World Sports Drug Agency'. *Performance Enhancement and Health, 2*(2), 80–83.

Mazanov, J. (2014). Drug control in sport: What, how and by whom? In B. Stewart, & M. Burke (Eds.), *Drugs and Sport: Writings from the Edge* (Chapter 2). Dry Ink Press: Melbourne, Australia.

Mazanov, J. (2016). Beyond anti-doping and harm minimisation: A stakeholder-corporate social responsibility approach to drug control for sport. *Journal of Medical Ethics, 42*(4), 220–223.

Mazanov, J., & McDermott, V. (2009). The case for a social science of drugs in sport. *Sport in Society, 12*(3), 276–295.

Mazanov, J., & Connor, J. (2010). Rethinking the management of drugs in sport. *International Journal of Sport Policy, 2*(1), 49–63.

Mazanov, J., Huybers, T., & Connor, J. (2012). Prioritising health in anti-doping: What Australians think. *Journal of Science and Medicine in Sport, 15*(5), 381–385.

Miah, A. (2004). *Genetically Modified Athletes: Biomedical Ethics, Gene Doping and Sport.* London: Routledge.

Milot, L. (2014). Ignorance, harm, and the regulation of performance-enhancing substances. *Harvard Journal of Sports and Entertainment Law, 5*(1), 91–146.

Pound, R., McLaren, R., & Younger, G. (2015). *Independent Commission Report #1.* Montreal: World Anti-Doping Agency.

Saugy, M., Lundby, C., & Robinson, N. (2014). Monitoring of biological markers indicative of doping: The athlete biological passport. *British Journal of Sports Medicine*, 48(10), 827–832.

Savulescu, J., Foddy, B., & Clayton, M. (2004). Why we should allow performance enhancing drugs in sport. *British Journal of Sports Medicine*, 38(6), 666–670.

Schneider, A. J. (2004). Privacy, confidentiality and human rights in sport. *Sport in Society*, 7(3), 438–456.

Sottas, P. E., Robinson, N., Rabin, O., & Saugy, M. (2011). The athlete biological passport. *Clinical Chemistry*, 57(7), 969–976.

Stewart. B., & Smith, A. (2014). *Rethinking Drugs in Sport*. Abingdon: Routledge.

Weatherburn, D. (2008). Dilemmas in harm minimisation. *Addiction*, 104(3), 335–339.

Chapter 13

Reflections on sport, drugs and integrity management

Drug control for sport remains a dynamic experiment in integrity management, with potent lessons for drug control, integrity management for sport and integrity management broadly. Given the evidence base built in previous chapters, this chapter should be taken as opinion rather than argument and evidence. It is a reflection, both from a scholarly and personal point of view, on sports, drugs and integrity management as set out in the previous chapters.

The lessons for drug control focus on whether anti-doping has created the opportunity to manage the integrity of sport. The lessons for integrity management as it relates to the sports sector more broadly provide some indication of which practices might be usefully adapted to other sectors, and which might need deeper consideration before implementation. I conclude the analysis with my personal insights having spent some time thinking about sport, drugs and integrity.

Has anti-doping worked?

Anti-doping was implemented on the belief drugs were a threat to the integrity of that which made sport intrinsically valuable. The convictions associated with those beliefs led to the creation of a policy juggernaut and an administrative dreadnaught. There is no question that anti-doping dominates drug control for sport, and is beginning to test the borders towards claiming policy space on drug control outside sport. Despite the status of the anti-doping policy, the essential question remains as to whether it has protected the integrity of sport.

Successes for anti-doping managing the integrity in sport

The anti-doping policy has been an outstanding success in three key ways. The first is that, with sport ceding drug control to external interests in the late twentieth century, anti-doping allowed first the Olympic movement and then the rest of sport to regain the initiative over the role of drugs in sport. As governments imposed incontestable coercive pressure on sport to take control of its own destiny in relation to drug control, sport also moved from being a victim to a powerful stakeholder in market contests between public and private sector interests around the role of drugs in society. From this point of view, anti-doping has allowed the development of trust among producers and consumers in a version of sport where the rules and values are at least well known, even if misunderstood. That is, anti-doping gives people a reason to trust that there is an attempt to protect the integrity of sport.

The second is that the anti-doping policy has created an elegant administrative structure that translates ideology into practice. Given the difficulties of policy implementation in both sport and other sectors, this achievement is an extraordinary feat of administration. The universality accorded to anti-doping means it can penetrate all areas of sporting practice, establishing a set of protocols that enables an administrative lingua franca across sport. This promotes trust in the production process by giving both producers and consumers confidence that there is a visible, active and powerful guardian of integrity for sport.

The third outstanding success of the anti-doping policy has been policy harmonisation. There are two levels of policy harmonisation that relate to anti-doping and integrity management. First, few policies can claim the level of international consensus enjoyed by anti-doping. Where international consensus can be difficult to achieve (e.g. climate change), so many countries and institutions signing up to the Code makes this a significant achievement in its own right. This sends a clear signal about the intent and strength behind the interest in protecting the integrity of sport. Second, despite policy variation remaining a feature of anti-doping practice, the nature and extent of that variation is less than might be expected. That the main features of the anti-doping policy (e.g. sanctions, therapeutic use exemption and out-of-competition testing) are implemented across signatories is a significant achievement despite the differences in practice that arise across jurisdictions. As implementation of anti-doping matures, experience should see variation decrease, or practices change where variation proves impossible to overcome. Implementation of any changes that do emerge will enjoy the benefits of both the administrative apparatus and experience, which should see a rapid and effective roll out that preserves both policy harmonisation and trust in the underlying processes. Thus, policy harmonisation remains a key part of any success anti-doping has in protecting the integrity of sport.

Failures for anti-doping managing the integrity in sport

As experience with the anti-doping policy grows, the unintended consequences of the policy that emerge suggest that anti-doping has failed to manage the integrity of sport effectively. Many of the failures are the result of apparent contradictions between the idealism of anti-doping and its practice.

There is no evidence that anti-doping has arrested drug-related harms in sport. The attempt to control so-called performance enhancing drugs has failed to diminish individual and institutional interest in consuming drugs in pursuit of sporting performance. Instead, anti-doping has shaped which drugs individuals and institutions pursue (e.g. contaminated supplements or experimental pharmaceuticals), and how they go about consuming them (e.g. unsupervised misuse or abuse). It is difficult to see how producers and consumers can trust sports production processes which sanction the consumption of drugs which may improve access to and experience of sport (e.g. testosterone replacement therapy), while promoting drugs which have demonstrably negative implications for both performance and health (e.g. alcohol).

An unintended consequence of anti-doping is the focus on a very narrow version of drug control at the expense of broader drug control. That is, the focus on doping risks detracts from the capacity to respond to integrity concerns arising from other drugs. The resourcing constraints associated with implementing anti-doping means under-resourcing to address other drug-related integrity threats; for example, being forced to invest in doping leaves sports programmes vulnerable to integrity threats from engagement with the e-cigarette, alcohol and supplements industries. This resourcing problem is only going to get worse as the costs of anti-doping compliance increase over time. Even though anti-doping may protect the integrity of sport from threats associated with doping, it has the capacity to make the integrity of sport vulnerable to threats from other drugs.

At the time of writing, the resourcing problem was also becoming an issue for poorer countries, with Kenya being asked to invest more heavily in anti-doping to meet its obligations to the international sporting community. Of course, Kenya may see nation building activities such as investing in education or health infrastructure as more of a priority than the integrity of sport. Again, this is likely to become more of an issue as the costs of anti-doping rise over time. Anti-doping is going to be unable to protect the integrity of sport if only wealthy countries can afford to do so.

The resourcing problem has already become manifest in terms of anti-doping being constructed to service the integrity needs of elite male sport, without regard for any other version of sport. For anti-doping to have legitimacy as drug control-led integrity management for sport, it needs to innovate such that the integrity of women's junior recreational sport is accorded the same status as elite men's professional sport. Without such a change, those charged with drug control-led integrity management send a signal that integrity is driven by commercial interests rather than any interest in the intrinsic value of sport.

The commercial interests driving integrity management may have also been entrenched from the outset of anti-doping. Anti-doping appears to serve institutional interests, demonstrated by its value as a business-to-business marketing device rather than an attempt to address integrity threats arising from drug misuse and abuse in sporting practice. The Spirit of Sport statement appears to have been designed to serve, or has been co-opted into serving, the interests of administrative convenience rather than serving as the moral basis for drug control-led integrity management. The hegemonic governance of anti-doping also appears to serve commercial interests, failing to address conflict of interest, transparency and democracy concerns. The most critical of these failures is the systematic exclusion of athletes from having an equal voice in matters that directly affect their lives, from the distressing and degrading experience of urinating in front of a stranger to being coerced into a surveillance system that prevents freedom of movement. Importantly, drug testing and surveillance constructed under the anti-doping policy may be better tolerated if they emerged from an organisation that included people whose lives are affected by the decisions.

Anti-doping-led integrity management for sport

While anti-doping appears to have had a significant impact as a method to manage the integrity of sport at the policy level, the capacity of anti-doping to protect the integrity of sport at any other level is less certain. Indeed, in attempting to manage integrity from one point of view, the resultant has been the creation of a set of new threats to the integrity of sport. On balance, then, it seems that the anti-doping policy experiment has failed to capitalise on the hard-won initiative with regards to managing integrity in sport.

Integrity management

The discussion of sport's attempt at drug control-led integrity management provides a basis to inform integrity management more broadly. This example becomes more important as the corporate social responsibility agenda gathers momentum across sectors, increasing demands upon organisations to do more than public relations, crisis management, or product harm marketing. The interest in, and therefore need to manage rather than respond to, integrity is growing.

It is perhaps a truism to say that integrity violations are inevitable, but it still needs to be said as a reminder for why integrity management is necessary. Another truism is that the introduction of integrity management is never going to prevent violations in trust relationships. One side of integrity management is establishing a set of mechanisms that allows an organisation or sector to identify threats that can be controlled, and to do something about them in terms of prevention or response. The other side to integrity management comes from completely unanticipated rules- or values-based violations of expectations.

Prior to the implementation of anti-doping, the Olympic movement approached drug control-led integrity management as a trivial symbolic exercise. They were caught unprepared by government demands they put administrative rigour behind the anti-doping policy. The lesson here is that discussions about integrity management need to be more than symbolic. The failure to engage with integrity management from the perspective of practice at the outset could see the attempt to preserve trust undermined by poorly specified practices. This is a sound reason why organisations need to be proactive with regards to integrity management.

Anti-doping presumed that there was a single 'right' version of sport, and that any other version of sport was 'wrong'. There was, unfortunately, a failure to integrate an understanding that justified the judgement beyond doping being 'wrong'. The consequence of the failure to develop a sophisticated moral basis for the policy was that it made it difficult to *manage* integrity adaptively. For example, a less certain moral approach may have seen sport able to exploit drugs more effectively to promote the integrity of sport (e.g. participation rates among older athletes) or to respond to other drug threats to the integrity of sport (e.g. tobacco, alcohol or supplements). Instead, the moral certainty saw sport implement blunt policy instruments on a narrow range of drugs, taking an approach that appeared to follow the aphorism that if you only have a hammer then everything starts to look like a nail.

Part of the specification of integrity comes from avoiding the trap of thinking that managers know best. That is, the people who produce or consume are likely to have a better understanding of rules- and values-based expectations, rather than those more remote to production or consumption. For example, integrity in line-production is likely to be very different to integrity among vice-presidents (individual *versus* institutional interests). As a result, integrity management may need to be constructed differently at different levels. In the event that a single universal policy is to be imposed, it is clear that views on integrity from across stakeholders are needed. That is, the assumption that a vice-president has special insight into what consumers think constitutes integrity in their industry is a dangerous one, and easily confirmed or discounted by asking some direct questions. Of course, it would be unreasonable to expect a stakeholder-driven approach to integrity management to anticipate all possibilities, but at least it is less likely to be beholden to a single dominant view.

A particularly important insight to be derived from anti-doping-led integrity management of sport is to separate policy from administration. That is, where anti-doping is an inflexible approach to integrity management, the administrative architecture that translates the policy into practice can be adapted to suit other policy approaches to integrity. The insight is therefore to avoid making the mistake of conflating the policy with the administration, such that while the content may be different the policy instruments can be largely the same. The most accessible method of achieving this is to exploit the policy instruments from human resource management to address integrity concerns. For example, innovations in integrity policy can take advantage of collective bargaining to structure democratic governance. Alternatively, employment contracts or performance management policies can be used to roll out integrity management initiatives more quickly.

Personal reflections on sports, drugs and integrity

My reflections take the form of critical reflexive practice, where I consider the pre- and post-effects of the project. Notably, one thing has remained constant for me throughout this project; my anxiety about the anti-doping policy.

Pre-project

When I started doing research on drugs in sport, it was with all the moral certainty that I see in so many others who declare their allegiance to 'drug-free sport'. The strength of my convictions came from Australia's devotion to the great sporting myth, and my belief in Australia as the greatest sporting nation on the planet.

When I started an academic career looking at the psychology of drug consumption, one of the first things my supervisor got into my head was that drugs can sometimes be right. We spent a lot of time talking about which of physical, mental, social or spiritual should be the focus for research seeking to protect 'health'. We also talked about the difference between drugs promoting and harming health. It should have been no surprise that when I applied such lines of thinking to drugs in sport the same answer seemed to fit the evidence. Drugs can help people access and enjoy the physical, mental, social and spiritual health benefits of sport, so that they can get the same things out of sport I did.

Of course, the anti-doping policy is antithetical to someone who takes this kind of view on drugs in sport. This is where my anxieties began to emerge; am I wrong to take this view? Everyone I have met who supports the anti-doping policy has firm convictions that drugs are anathema to the integrity of sport. They are genuine, passionate and well-intentioned people who can see how doping harms the individuals, teams and organisations that make up modern sport. Their certainty makes me wonder about my own views, and so I keep going back to the arguments and evidence to try to figure out whether, in good conscience, I should keep thinking about drugs in sport as 'good' or 'bad'; whether I should keep questioning or add my support to anti-doping.

Some years ago, I had a conversation with a very prominent figure in anti-doping. The conversation went something along the lines that they believed drug-free sport was worth fighting for. I surprised both of us by asking why their belief in drug-free sport was worth more than my idea that drugs have an important role in sport, why they were allowed to impose their desire for drug-free sport on me rather than the other way around. In essence, I was asking why their definition of integrity in sport was worth defending. There was no easy answer to this question for either of us, but it got me thinking about the question of drug control as integrity management for sport.

Things all changed when I became a father, and the question of whether I would let my kids play sport came up. I started looking into the implications of anti-doping for children. When I realised what a drug test would mean for my children, my anxiety about anti-doping returned. Then I started thinking through what it meant for young women. It raised all sorts of questions for me about what people were willing to do to each other to protect the 'integrity of sport'. This started bringing up the questions about integrity management addressed throughout this book.

Post-project

Four chapters in particular shaped my thinking. The first was thinking through the implications of integrity management for human resource management. The standard approaches to integrity management reflect conventional thinking, something which is easy to do and intuitively linked to results. The implication for me was the ongoing disconnection between evidence and professional practice, which seems to be characteristic of integrity management. Rather than draw on evidence, integrity management, like other forms of management, seems to prefer to draw on what feels right rather than take advantage of the available evidence. While the recommendations may be more difficult to achieve, I have never seen something being hard as a reason to discount a course of action. Of course, others may take a different view.

Working towards a business ethics rather than sports ethics approach to drug control for sport was formative. The key insight I drew from writing about business ethics was the realisation why people get so upset when I contradict their beliefs about the role of drugs in sport. For example, it was a revelation understanding that those who believe in anti-doping see people like me as morally immature. This revelation has helped me to appreciate their point of view a lot better, and to stop taking their vigorous defence of their preferred version of sport quite so personally. In doing so,

I recognised that trying to work out what we mean by integrity in sport is trickier than most of us realise. Ending up with anti-doping may have simply been the least diabolical approach when sport was wrestling with these sorts of issues. That being said, the role of sport in society has changed since sport first started wrestling with ideas of integrity and drugs, and it needs a rethink.

Exploring governance improved my understanding of why anti-doping is structured the way it is. Anti-doping really is a marvellous piece of systemic governance, and I can see why some of my colleagues get very excited when talking about it. The corollary to this is that it makes the failures at the organisational level much worse. It is almost like the architects of anti-doping spent all their time worrying about the UN and the IOC, and forgot about whether it was actually going to work for athletes and support personnel. It reminds me of the sage advice that Evil Overlords should retain a five-year-old child to point out the flaws in their insanely convoluted schemes to catch the Good Guy. Perhaps those in charge of drug control in sport need to stop thinking about sport at the institutional level and take advice on what integrity in sport means from people who actually engage in play, game and sport.

The fourth highly influential chapter for me was my examination of non-elite and non-male sport. While I had suspicions along these lines before I started this project, spending the effort to look into those suspicions deepened them into strong concerns. Any organisation that thinks it is okay to conduct a witnessed drug test of a pre-adolescent child because they 'might' do something wrong has to have a good long hard look at proportionality. I am unsure how drug testing a child protects the integrity of the 100 metres men's final at the Summer Olympics. I am also yet to be convinced that drug testing a child does much more than potentially terrifying the child into compliance or out of sport. Having said that, knowledge is power, and I think I might be ready to let my kids play sport, with a few amendments to the membership agreement ...

Conclusions on drugs, sport and integrity

My reflections on this project lead me back to my view that we need to have rigorous drug control for sport. I am yet to be dissuaded from my view that anti-doping serves neither the integrity of athletes nor the integrity of sport. If anything, this project has heightened my concerns that anti-doping impugns the dignity of athletes without really doing much to improve the integrity of sport or those associated with sport. By respecting athlete dignity as the centre of practice, I remain optimistic that drug control can contribute to the integrity of sport without compromising the intrinsic value of sport – the people who want to share their deep passion for playing the games they love.

Index

Page numbers in *italics* denote tables.